W9-CQR-597

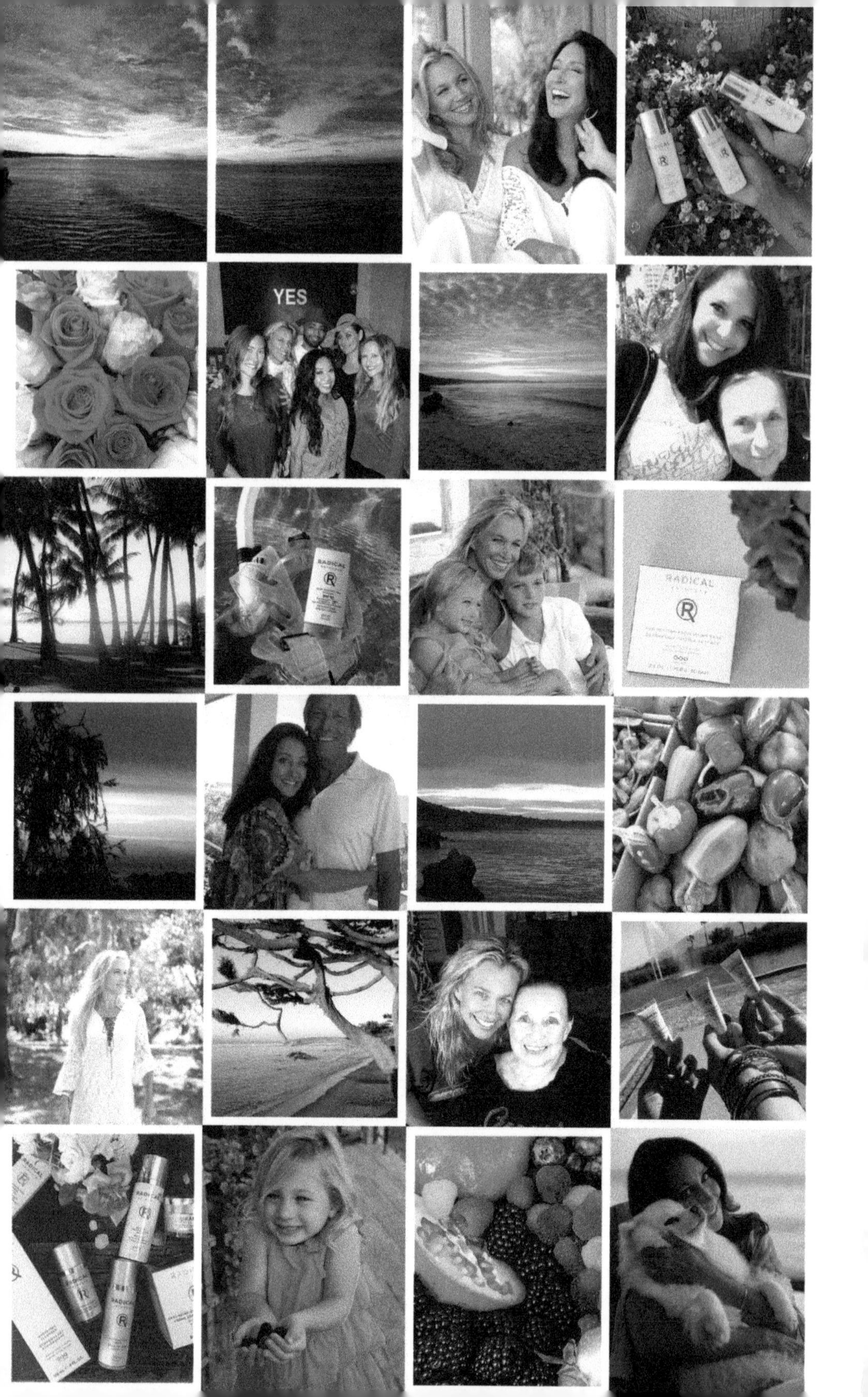
YES
RADICAL

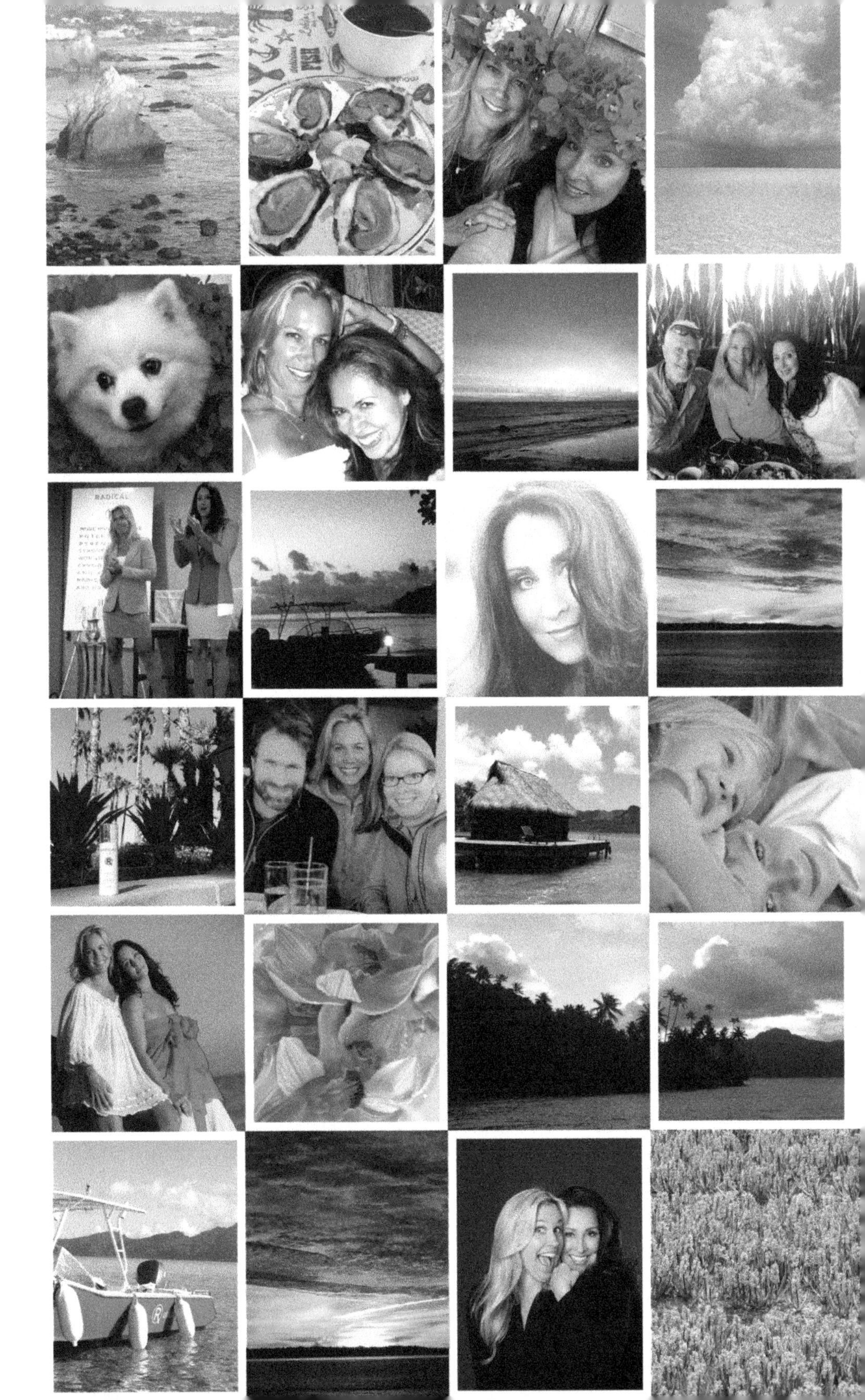
RADICAL

GET RADICAL

Secrets to Creating a Life You Love

RACHEL & LIZ EDLICH

CREATORS OF RADICAL SKINCARE, DAUGHTERS OF RICHARD F. EDLICH, MD, PHD

Published by
Hasmark Publishing
judy@hasmarkpublishing.com

First Edition, 2016

Editor: Justin Spizman
www.JustinSpizman.com

Cover Design:
Patti Knoles
www.VirtualGraphicArtsDepartment.com

Erika Dang
www.erikadang.com

Layout: Ginger Marks
www.DocUmeantDesigns.com

Front cover photo by Greg Gorman
www.gormanphotography.com

ISBN-13: 978-1-988071-12-1
ISBN-10: 1988071127

DEDICATION

We dedicate this book to our friends, family, mentors and those who have touched us throughout our life journey. Your love and kindness are reflected in these pages and are the source of our passion that compelled us to share your inspiration with others.

FOREWORD

GO FOR IT: GET RADICAL

It is as simple as that. Most of us don't do what we want. We do what we think will keep us in place, or just occasionally stretch ourselves a little further than the norm. But if we are going after what we want, we have got to be radical. We've got to get out of the box. We have to decide, almost instantly, to flip the light switch and shed light on those elements of life that hold us back. To be radical, the key ingredient is to make the decision that's the way we are going to live. Once we make that decision, we can already begin to see the difference. That's an important step to getting what we want: making the decision and using our will to accomplish it.

Liz and Rachel will help you create the energy you need to be radical. They will help you to become mentally strong and absolutely directed. They offer you a prescription that is digestible and can position both you and your life for great levels of success. But you have to be disciplined. Discipline is giving yourself a command and then following it. Radical is not easy. Radical is not for lightweights. You've got to be ready. And the beautiful part about this is that as you work at it you'll find your strength grows to be stronger, and stronger, and stronger. And that is when you are living the life you really want to live. Radical is having a mission. It's knowing where you are going. It's being fulfilled. It's living a meaningful life.

Take a look around. People constantly surround us. Those that know us are used to looking at us in a certain way and knowing exactly the way we are. But when we get radical, it is like we create a new person, one that may be unfamiliar to some, but is the absolute best version of ourselves. Sometimes we are the only one that sees it—it could be invisible to many. And they might think we are just a little bit crazy. But eventually they will come around as well, and realize that we are radical, and we want to be proud of the fact. We can have it all. We can visualize a life filled with abundance and success.

We are all aware that time on this beautiful earth is limited, so it should be a good time. You are going to have a good time when you've got a real good reason to get out of bed in the morning and make it happen. That's what a radical person does – that's how he or she lives. You cannot go by the norm. You cannot let precedent control your decisions. Start to understand who you are. The radical person is independent. The radical individual is courageous. They go where they want to go even though they've never been there. Fear doesn't stop them. You see, radical individuals have fear, but they don't let it get in their way. They go where most people have never been. And that's what makes them radical. It's a beautiful concept when you really understand it.

So, what are you waiting for? A radical person is a super-serious student. They are always studying something they don't understand, because they want to gain a better understanding of how to improve. They realize understanding only comes one way – through dedicated study. They understand that understanding is the polar opposite to doubt and worry. So, when doubt and worry strike, they know it's because there's something they don't understand and they start studying. They eliminate the doubt and the worry, which lead to fear, and they go to understanding, which leads to faith and expression. They're creative individuals. Together, through reading this book, we are going to create a radical future for you.

There is no reason why we can't all be radical. I want to be more radical. Liz and Rachel are two radical women. They get it. They talk the talk and then thunderously walk the walk. You can hear them coming a mile away. And once they get here, their presence is encompassing, invigorating, and absolutely welcoming. Their radical journey is a special one and I am thankful they are willing to share it with you. I appreciate the prescription they created and use it in my own life. Even though I think I am a pretty radical guy, I became more radical as I read this book. It pushed me, challenged me, and awoke my senses to be present in life and radical in my journey. But for Liz and Rachel, I would not be nearly as radical as I am today. I attribute a portion of my growth to their personal journey. They care deeply, share openly, and are truly difference makers in the game of life.

This book is for those of you that awake each day and want to brighten the world. It takes great energy and inspiration to do so. But if you cannot always find the inspiration and direction to be a game-changer, then get ready to feel an overwhelming amount of hope to find your passion path. Passion, purpose, and complete health await you. You have much of what is needed, but now you can sprinkle in a little bit of a radical approach to create a limitless life filled with your heart's desire. You may feel numb and have forgotten to dream. But Liz and Rachel will help you believe and have daily passion. Beyond these pages are the tools to turn the pages in your life. With each page you'll gain momentum that will propel you forward to reach your goals.

This book will give you the radical access you'll need to bring home what you truly desire. The love you want, the life you deserve, and the resources to get you there just require a Radical Yes. So buckle your seat belt because Liz and Rachel are determined friends that will see you through the journey. They inspire me and will inspire you to live outside the box and get radical. So get ready to laugh on, love on, and embrace all of the success in areas that really matter. Ask yourself before turning to the next page: What radically rocks my world?

You want to be radical? I sure hope you do. I am radical. Liz is radical. Rachel is radical. We can be radical together. So go for it: Get radical.

Bob Proctor

ACKNOWLEDGMENTS

A VERY RADICAL THANK YOU!

Get Radical is the culmination of intense focus, late nights and weekends to communicate a lifetime of valuable lessons learned through some of the most amazing friends, family and visionaries. It was part of our legacy and dream to share the lessons in this book with people worldwide in hopes of making a radical difference in their lives.

We would first like to thank our wonderfully inspiring parents. Without their love and devotion and creating the radical roots for us to grow from, we would not have been driven by such unbridled passion and purpose to share our story with you.

To Dad: although you are not with us today, your spirit encouraged us to say the Radical Yes to this challenge, like you did during your life.

And to our Mother Carol: who would weep with joy and tears of pride upon reading this, we hope that when you turn the pages it breathes life and memory back into that kind and gentle soul who dances in the rain.

Our brother Richard and his beautiful wife Patricia: we thank you for grounding us in the simple pleasures and traditions of family as well a demonstrating the gift of giving and growing as a committed couple.

From Rachel: to my beautiful children Forrest and Sophia. Thank you for keeping me young and reminding me about the important things in life. You allow me to experience unconditional love and raw laughter with the innocence that inspires me to be a kid again.

From Liz: to my wonderful husband Dale, whose support and love allows me to go after my dreams and express the passion and purpose that resides within. And to our son Matthew: who gave me the journey of motherhood and the gift of pride and the opportunities to share with him the secret that daschunds can fly. My nephew Forrest and niece Sophia, who keep it real and grounded; I love you to the moon and back again.

Of course there are always the individuals that see your immense possibility even when you find the challenge too overwhelming and the mountain too steep. We would like to thank Bob Proctor for his generous teachings, coaching and unwavering belief in what it means to be Radical. His wisdom graces the pages of our lives and his words echo in our mind as we walk through life sharing his teachings that so empowered us. Our friend Cynthia Kersey, who stood fast that this book should be our journey and coached us step by step in the process. Don Miguel Ruiz, who years ago said that we should write a book that expressed our *Authentic Self* and no matter that we told him it would take too much time, cost too much money, and it was just too much of everything, he just smiled and said that you will write that book.

We thank our Radical family of friends, partners and ambassadors who have shone their light on this journey, giving us encouragement, strength, laughter and support. Our worldwide Sisters and Misters on a mission that have worked tirelessly to take us, Radical Skincare and our Radical message of empowerment around the world helps to prove that it truly takes a village. Thanks to Greg Gorman, Sandra James, Valerie Plotnikova, Leah-Vail Soloff, Erin Davis, Adriane Boat, Erika Dang, Marc Benhamou, Marie-Camille Auber, Susie Jones, Frankie Neal, Danette Eilenberg, Samantha Hart, Emma Elliot, Rowley Weeks, Jeff Stroud, Brad Wayment, Tina Tomson, Martha McCully, Katrin Fulluck, Sylvaine Falque, Genvieve Du Parc, Franziska and Rudolf Kaelin, Ted Edlich, Emma Louise Haswell, Katie England, Hanna Smith, Kimberly Gray, Erik Makowski, Kasia Komorowicz, Vesa Kalho, Hofit Golan, Tracey Woodward, Caroline Hirons, Sian Sutherland, Marie Rose Tricon, Fabienne Sisco, Sarah Griffiths, Kathy Laura Makowski, Samios Family and Zach Samios, Gerry Shillings (BC Fulfillment), Gregory Watson, Jennifer and Jason Gilbert, Olga and Sam Crawford, John Gustafson, Freyja Barker, Kevin Harris, Bertie Kearsey, Barbara Devorzon, Yvette Mimeux, Melanie Griffith, Goldie Hawn, Sabina Morales, Tracy Ryan-Johnson, Marcy Jo Anderson, Dawn Lee Johnson, Rhonda Conroy and Peter Anton, Cynthia La Roche, Shawn Taddey, Dodee Coble Smith, Dionea Orcini, Howard Ruby, Aunt

Nicky Edlich and Aunt Karen Weiss, Silvia Rodriguez, Willie Perez, Moses Dean, Dyan Cannon, Monique Nichols, Dorotha Rey, Eva Vapori, Ethel Tuterai LeDoux, Vai and Tyrone Tucker, Bettina O'neil, Christine and George Moarii, Virginie and Tama Castagnoli, Eileen Bossuot-Surleau, Tracy Giles, Princess Sophie Audouin Mamikonian, Tammy Strome, Larry Willis, Kasey Walker, Malika Wiezbowski, Gina LeCabe, Mareva Georges, Ileana Platt, Shirley Sherman, Maria Price, Mike Price, Ali and Paige Price, Sally and Donald Ratner, India Martin, Rodger Linse Andrea and Ann King, Lisa Gordon, Dolores Granato, Miss Glo, Patti Reilly, Sabina Morales, Cindy Anderson, Sherry Williams, Lesley Rogers, Ruben Torres, Nasra Atar, Amra Hajdarevic, Baroness Patricia Scotland, Lavinia Errico, Clever Zulu, Dan Buettner, Tori Cowen, Stephanie Cooper, Tippi Hedren, Dino Buccola, Jaicey Harding, Deepak Chopra, Master Stephen Co, Ale Armas and Doug Deluca, and a big thank you to our incredible retail partners around the world, QVC and our Radical sister QVC hosts.

Our business Angels and friends, Alfred Cheng, Raymond Cheng, David Torjman, Maurice Marciano, Paul Marciano, Todd Kesselman, Ariel and Karine Ohana, Patrick Bousquet Chavanne, Paul Henri Duillet, Jean Paul Imbert, Clifton Tan, Bernard Gaude, Didier Picard, Michel Grunberg, David Peteler, Seth Bogner, Ivan and Carmen Sotomayer, Gene Fina, Richard Krajchek and Daphne Deckers, Victor Sturing.

A special thanks to cutting edge science and the formulation that has gone into creating Radical Skincare. Without this life-changing discovery and proprietary Trylacel technology, we would not have taken this Radical Journey. The scientific minds of Lionel De Benetti and James Wilmott as well as the manufacturing genius of Alban Muller and team of Alban Muller International and Doug and David Johnson and team at Cosmetic Laboratories, thank you for going above and beyond in your creativity.

This book would not have seen the light of day but for Peggy McColl, Judy O'Beirn and the creative and heartfelt expression and editing of Justin Spizman. Their partnership has been a true gift.

And to all of you that we have met on our journey in seventeen countries over the past four years, thank you for the special and inspiring moments that we shared with one another. It is because of you that we were inspired to write this book.

A PERSONAL NOTE

A personal note to our sisters and misters on a mission:

A there was a time when building a skincare company was our first and foremost goal. It was our purpose; it was our calling. It was what we thought of as we dozed off at night, and what excited us enough to forego the snooze button in the early morning hours. We lived it, we breathed it, and eventually, we created it. John Lennon inspired us by stating, "There's nowhere you can be that isn't where you're meant to be." We truly believe we were meant to develop this company.

We spent numerous years pioneering, developing, and perfecting a skincare line that was strong enough to fight the signs of aging and gentle enough to be used on sensitive skin. The journey to creating our luxury skincare company, *Radical Skincare*, was long in the making, but absolutely worth the wait. It certainly didn't happen overnight, and also would not have been possible without the Radical innovators and supporters along the way. These kindred souls made taking those leaps of faith just a little bit easier. Their stories and sustenance have served as a perpetual source of inspiration for us.

But something special and unexpected happened along the way. We started our journey destined to build an amazing skincare line, but began to realize that the principles and fundamentals we applied to our business were actually applicable to bettering our lives. So we started looking at things a little bit more radically. Think for a minute about your skincare regime as a metaphor for your life. Similar to creating a healthy and nourishing skincare regiment, each of our lives can benefit from fundamental practices like removing belief systems that are outdated and that dull your true beauty while inhibiting your radiant nature. Sounds a lot like exfoliating, right? Or how about clearing your mind and creating a blank palette and a receptive canvas to eventually produce amazing results in your life. That may remind you of cleansing. Finally, what about the act of nourishing your inner fabric with people that support your goals and future success? That would ring of moisturizing.

The list goes on and on. From our perspective, the essential behaviors supporting a healthy and active skincare routine parallel the components that sustain a flourishing and thriving life. And we are confident after reading this book, you will not only agree, but will also implement these practices into your own skincare routine and your own life.

For us, living a *Radical* life evolved through developing and growing our skincare line. But it has quickly become second nature. We are the daughters of Dr. Richard F. Edlich MD.PHD, world-renowned Professor of Plastic Surgery. Working in our father's lab before the age of ten and at the University of Virginia Burn Unit, we were exposed to the science of skin rejuvenation and wound repair at extreme levels. Our business started with a challenge to chemists and scientists to create the most powerful anti-aging solution that could still be used on sensitive skin.

In our small lab, we created sample bottles, which were labeled with a magic marker and used on our own faces and the faces of our friends. The results were radical. We started our company to solve a problem within our own lives, but we quickly found we were not alone. As of the publishing of this book, we have taken Radical Skincare from two stores in the United States to over 800 prestigious stores in fifteen countries in just under four years: Radical growth from some radical women.

True to our commitment to put the money in the bottle and not into advertising or paying for expensive packaging or celebrities, Radical Skincare has grown organically and through word of mouth. Having created the strongest skincare line that can be used on even the most sensitive skins, we take skincare with a message of inspiration and empowerment to create Radical results.

As you can tell, *Radical* is an important word to us. But what does it really mean?

As a noun, it is defined as a person who holds or follows strong convictions or extreme principles.

As an adjective, it is considered as extreme, especially in regards to change from accepted or traditional forms.

These definitions excite us. They make us feel unique and different. But what they really do is inspire us to not only understand, but also evaluate and consider what living a Radical life looks like.

Radical means remaining persistent when it's easier to quit.

Radical means not being afraid of failing, but terrified of not trying.

Radical means turning a challenge into an opportunity.

Radical means making a difference by being the difference.

Radical means changing yourself so you can change others.

Our definition of Radical is continually evolving. As we meet our current goals and constantly strive to set fresh ones, it takes on new and exciting meaning in our quest for a life that is filled with happiness, fulfillment, and unparalleled success. Sound intriguing? Well we are confident that our experience can inspire you to do the same. A radical life is a special and empowering one that reverberates at a high frequency. It is vibrant, colorful, and bright. We think it's pretty cool. It illuminates the path for others and shines true on those in need.

Together, we can take the principles that built our company and apply them to reinvigorate, refresh, and rejuvenate your own life. We hope that this book will help move you closer towards creating a Radical life that excites you, fulfills you, nurtures you, and empowers you. It is possible to love your skin and your life. You just have to be Radical in your approach.

With Radical Regards,

Liz Edlich

Rachel Edlich

Chapter 1
RADICAL BEGINNINGS

Do you have a word? Think of that one word. The one you go back to time and time again. It may comfort you. It could inspire you. Maybe it motivates you. But we all have that one word. We say it too much. We think about it all the time. It is the reason why we stay up at night and wake up in the morning. We identify with it more than people may even recognize. It could be our motto. Maybe it is our slogan.

That one word.

It is powerful and enormously exciting. It ignites our life and fires us up. The heat it creates warms others. They can feel it, even if they are unable to identify it. It ushers in happiness and deflects sadness.

Just one word.

No matter what people tell you, words and ideas can change the world. They have certainly changed ours. There was a time when our path was unclear. We can still identify the time when we had more problems than solutions. We couldn't identify our own adage. We weren't totally lost, but we weren't found either.

We were looking for that right word.

John F. Kennedy reminded us "as we express our gratitude, we must never forget that the highest appreciation is not to utter words, but to live by them." Special things happen when words are driven by passion and purpose. Lives can be changed when words are injected with meaning. As these words are then transformed into action, the result is an unprecedented level of success. For us, our journey started with identifying one word that truly made the difference.

We all have words. What is the word that occurs as a theme in your life?

Your word may be passion, love, kindness, giving, purpose, family, maybe even commitment. This book is about our special word – one we think that by the end of the journey, you will also resonate with. It is about a word that changed our lives; a word we believe will change yours. In fact, it became our personal axiom. It is an adjective, noun, and verb that we use to describe all facets of our own life. This word jumpstarted our business, inspired our life, and is now the word we put before others, above others, and instead of others.

That word is *radical.* It describes who we are, how we live, and what we strive for. Transitioning to a radical life took time. As you'll see in the forthcoming pages, our journey was at times anything but radical. While we came from unique and exciting roots, we faced a lot of adversity early on. But we were always grounded in the notion that there was something bigger and something resounding about a life that seemed more like destiny than reality.

That destiny led us to begin the process of writing this book, and to use our journey through life to support your journey. As sisters, our journeys are distinctly different, but also strikingly similar. This book is our story, our collective and individual thoughts, the story of friends and others that we have met along the way. This is our radical attempt to authentically share with you the education we garnered that made the difference for us and for the thousands of people we have coached and mentored.

Depending on the moment and the radical lesson at hand, one of us may take the lead while the other provides the support. We each have our own perspectives, journeys, and experiences, and while they have all intersected throughout our lives, those lenses are special and unique to each one of us. Throughout this book we will share our collective thoughts as well as our unique stories and perspectives.

IT STARTED WITH A RADICAL MOMENT

We grew up believing we could – and would – do whatever we set our mind to.

Believing in yourself comes naturally when you have parents who would not quit…

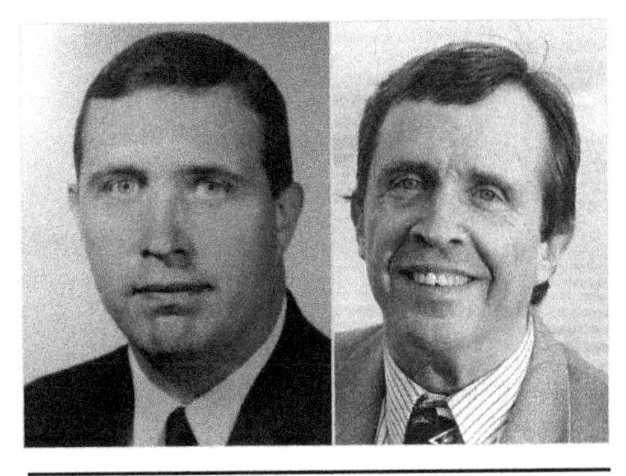

Our Dad

Our father grew up on the lower East side of New York City and graduated high school at the age of fifteen, college at eighteen, and medical school at the age of twenty-two. His rapid acceleration through traditional education and early departure from home was largely driven by his need to escape his drug addicted mother and somewhat abusive and absentee father. Through Dad's quest for survival, he became a brilliant reconstructive plastic surgeon who started the burn unit at the University of Virginia, created Steri-Strips (dissolvable sutures), and served as the head of Emergency Medical Services for Virginia. Sadly, life presented Dad with another challenge: He developed multiple sclerosis and was confined to a wheelchair for the last half of his career and his life. But that didn't stop him. He published more than three thousand peer-reviewed journal articles through dictation while being immobile from the neck down.

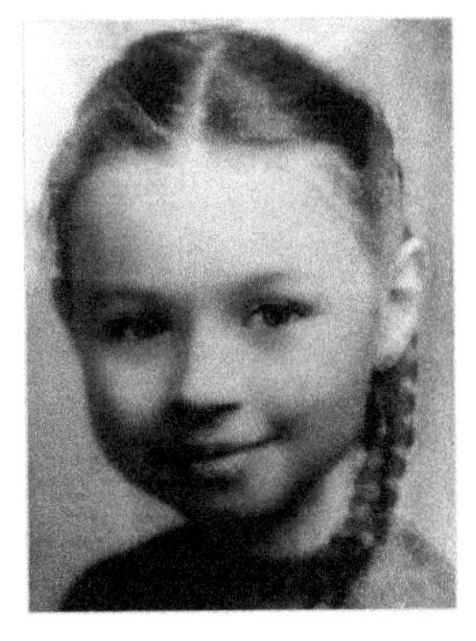

Mom at age 12

Our mother grew up with very little. Her mom worked at Kodak and baked, and her dad serviced heating and air conditioners. She spent her childhood in Rochester, New York and attended Catholic school. She was on a clear path to be a nun. She had a dream to be on Broadway, but without ever having voice or acting lessons, the odds of her achieving her dream were slim. One day she made a radical decision to move to New York City anyway, and after tireless days and months of auditions and singing in nightclubs, she landed the role of Maria in *West Side Story* on Broadway.

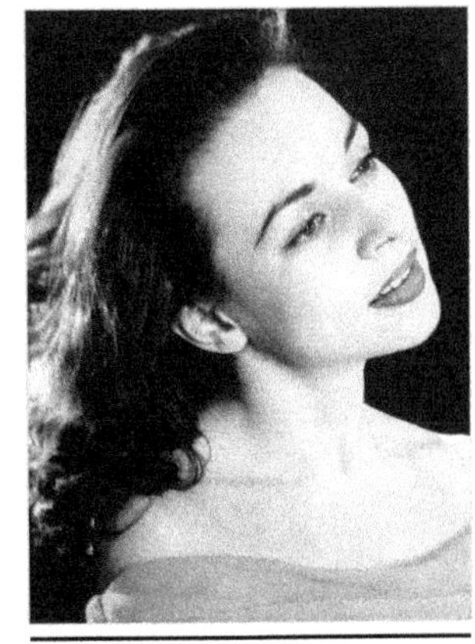

Our Mom in West Side Story

So we have "you can do it" blood pumping through our veins. Like our parents, we come from a complicated childhoods. Growing up with a hard driving perfectionist father with MS, and a mother suffering from anxiety and working to raise their three kids wasn't at all easy. Through a winding and bumpy road we've been blessed to enjoy successful careers while working together in the skincare industry for nearly twenty years. With a client list that included numerous celebrities, influencers, and everyday women across the country, we created quite a fulfilling career for ourselves.

BUT THEN SOMETHING HAPPENED THAT ATE AWAY AT OUR CONFIDENCE . . .

Liz: As with most really big opportunities, there was a defining flash of inspiration. For us, it was a radical moment that changed the environment of our own lives. We still refer to it as a perfect storm. After being immersed in the skincare industry in Los Angeles for over fifteen years and creating more than one hundred products for celebrities and women all over the world, our business became very personal when we experienced our own set of problematic skin issues.

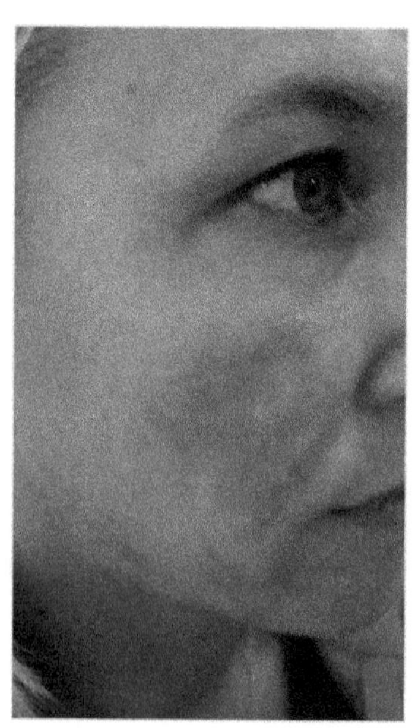

Founder Rachel Edlich with Rosacea

After having her second child, Rachel developed a very aggressive form of Rosacea. She had red bumps all over her face and was completely inflamed. She was quickly diagnosed and prescribed three different types of medication. The doctors told her that she would take these meds for the remainder of her adult life. For someone who had beautiful skin for years, this was a devastating situation. Aside from physical manifestations – the burning skin and red bumps that were lurking below the surface and ready to emerge depending on the day – Rachel was left feeling self-conscious and depressed, and had lost a real sense of confidence.

RADICAL *fact*

It is estimated that sixteen million Americans have rosacea! [1]

Simultaneously, I was experiencing my own set of issues and was joined by a chorus of girlfriends singing the same tune. After crossing the age of forty-five, I realized gravity was real and noticed wrinkles, loss of elasticity, and an overall sagging of my skin. It was as if I woke up one morning, looked in the mirror, and saw a different person staring back at me. Overnight the aging fairies held a conference and said, "Girlfriend, you've had it way too easy for far too long. It's time for you to wake up and smell the coffee and see what forty-five years of wear and tear looks like." On top of it, I felt the impact of my hormones changing. You know the feeling, and if you don't, stay tuned. Weight gain, dry skin and nails, mood swings, fatigue, and an overall sense of "now what?"

For the first time in our lives, after being in the business of beauty, we felt a sense of helplessness and frankly hopelessness. Nothing we tried actually worked and made a real difference. It was hard for Rachel to look at herself in the mirror. For me, the mirror only seemed to magnify all the changes in my face, body, and skin. Our minds began to fill with negative self-talk.

But then something our father had said to us countless times started to play in our minds: *To be the difference you must make the difference.*

Remembering his words prompted us to look for a solution. We were conditioned since we were kids that when the going gets tough, the tough get going.

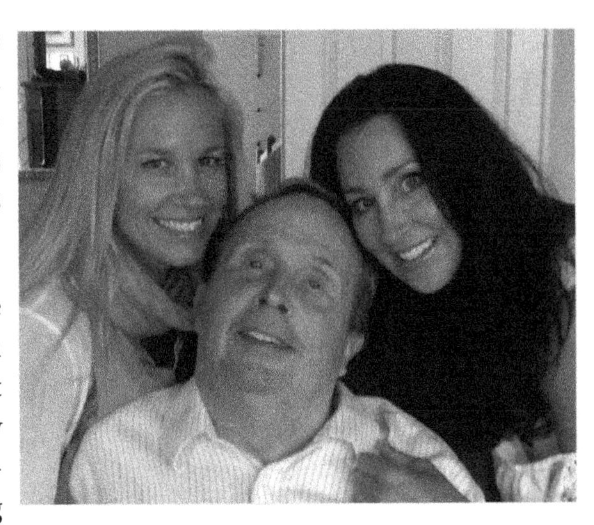

Rachel & Liz Edlich with their Father, Dr. Edlich

Together, we began the journey to find a solution for our skin problems, but in the end this journey became so much more – it became more fulfilling than we ever dreamed. Our challenges inspired us to find and craft a transformational prescription for skin, as well as a potent prescription for a radical life.

Dedicated to a sisterly solution, it was imperative to embrace and address both of our issues. We turned to chemists and scientists and challenged them to create the most powerful anti-aging solution, one that could defy gravity for me and at the same time heal Rachel's sensitive skin. After two years of trial and error, we developed a proprietary technology that delivered what we wanted. The results spoke for themselves. A lab compared our formulas to numerous leading skincare brands, and the potency results were unbeatable.

What we created in our little plastic lab sample bottles, and labeled with a magic marker – serum, moisturizer, eye – radically changed our skin. We both had almost immediate radical transformations. For the first time in my career in the beauty industry, I was stopped on the street and asked what I used on my skin. Friends started calling and asking what I put in the little plastic bottles that I gave them as party favors at lunch. Their skin never looked so good. Meanwhile, Rachel's Rosacea cleared and friends called her with similar problems, hoping she'd share her solution.

Just as our father transformed the landscape of medicine, we felt compelled to share our findings worldwide to make a radical difference in skincare and ultimately in lives. This was our radical moment. We didn't totally understand it at the time, but we had identified two mega-problems, and with care and great attention to detail, found a radical solution to both of them.

RADICAL *fact*

Many who suffer from skin conditions report experiencing low self-esteem, lack of confidence, anxiety, and depression.[2]

We took the challenge and created a radical solution. Then it hit us: The principles we used to change our skin were in essence the same fundamental principles we used in our everyday lives. This process of transforming the landscape of skincare could also be shared with others to inspire them to do the same!

Radical Skincare has not only transformed our skin, it has transformed our lives. And now, using skincare as a metaphor for life, we're helping others around the world to do the same. So how do you do that? How do you apply a winning formula to your life? And how can the simple act of using your skincare routine morning and night anchor and remind you of these key steps?

Using skincare as a metaphor for life is the easy part. It is incorporating key ingredients and mastering the process that is the hard part. Once you do, we call that a prescription. You may be reading this and saying to yourself, "Skincare as a metaphor for life? That's a stretch."

Not really. Take a simple example: What are some of the things that hold us back, disempower us, and stop us from doing and getting what we want out of life?

The answer is our past, our paradigms, and our negative self-talk that runs amuck in our minds. But what would we all like? We would all like to be free from a past that doesn't serve us, free from paradigms or conditioning that keeps us stuck and delivers results that are not in alignment with our heart's desires. And after cleansing this negativity away, we would all like a mental reboot to replace negative self-talk with empowering conversations that help us win.

RADICAL *fact*

More than 50 percent of the population is over the age of fifty, which means so is their skin![3]

Our commitment is to share with you the ingredients and the process needed to create your dreams. Just as there is a formula for creating amazing skincare products, there's a formula for creating a life you love. You might just need a pound of passion, a cup of purpose, or a spoonful of focus. We know that we can change the complexion of your skin. Our real personal payoff will be to know that we have changed the complexion of your life.

Chapter 2: WHAT IS RADICAL?

The most logical place for us to start is by defining the star of the show. The word radical has previously been tied directly to the feminist movement. But we are pro-people, cross cultural, and are building a paradigm of inclusion and not exclusion. The word radical can have a polarizing energy, one that fights against something or for something from an extreme point of view.

To that end, we believe in becoming radical in a way that goes to extremes to deliver life-changing skincare and lessons that break through the barriers and cross borders. Part of that journey resides in the notion that we will never accept the unacceptable, and will always strive to provide something better for the world. Radical embraces all that is possible and transcends boundaries to deliver honesty, potency, and performance to empower your skin and your life, and help you build *Radical Results* and nothing less.

We didn't always fully understand what the word radical meant. So before we adopted it as our mantra, our mission, and the name for our new business, we took the time to dive deeper into the meaning of the word radical and compile a list of words that go hand in hand.

That original list of words included:

- Unconventional
- Out of the box
- Against the grain
- Extreme
- Essential
- Basic
- Profound
- Deep-rooted
- Pervasive
- Revolutionary
- Evolutionary
- Fundamental
- Roots

These were just a few of the words we scribbled down when we were playing a radical word-game. But over time this one word has garnered a much greater meaning than even we originally anticipated. And our list has grown along with it.

Rachel: When we first started the company, radical had a connotation of really going against the grain and not conforming. That was what I thought of first when I heard the word radical. Now what I hear so much from others is that radical is "pushing one's individuality." From a traditional sense, it's calling me to live outside the lines. Living outside what's expected and not conforming to what you might think is the way to do something.

Liz: For me, when I look at the traditional definition of radical, it stands for "at the root of." It also means extreme. So when someone says rad or radical, of extreme sports or people who are being extreme in their views and in their actions, the word radical has a past and a legacy. Our definition is different from that. Our definition embraces the extreme nature of going above and beyond, about not taking no for an answer, about not accepting the unacceptable, about pushing barriers and boundaries, and going beyond the ordinary to reach levels of extraordinary.

RADICAL IS STRONG

As an adjective, radical is "relating or affecting the fundamental nature of something, far-reaching, thorough, complete, total, comprehensive, exhaustive, sweeping, extensive, across the board, profound, rigorous."

But for us, it transcends the dictionary definitions. For a long time radical was not something we defined, but something we felt. It was not a word but rather a way of life. And now, for you, radical can be a conduit for something bigger. Radical can inject passion, fuel purpose, and inspire you to create something greater.

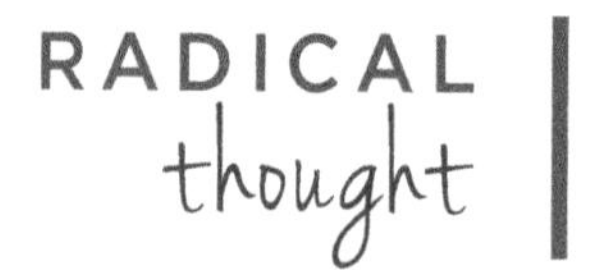

Radical is a lifestyle, a way of showing up in the world.

Radical means more honesty, more potency and more performance. It is really going above and beyond. As we're thinking it through, radical is having really strong values. It is driven through autonomy. It is grounded in empowerment, going above and beyond, and never taking *no* for an answer. It is uncompromising, maximum performance, tenacity, persistence, and passion. Radical is powerful results and nothing less.

We'll share with you the radical roadmap to get you to your preferred destination, but like anything you must be invested, engaged, and do the work.

Much like our Radical Skincare line, our definition for living and creating a radical life is fundamentally grounded in a harmonious blend of potent ingredients. Ingredients that add up to a radical life.

Just like baking a cake or creating a skincare line, you can incorporate ingredients in your life at different levels or amounts. A little too much of this or not enough of that and your cake, your skincare line, or your life will simply fall flat. It may also lack flavor if you forget the sugar, or lack moisture if there's not enough eggs or wet ingredients, and may come off as doughy or even burnt if you apply too much heat. Cake, skincare, and life: All the same. Success in each of these endeavors can be measured in the synchronistic mixture of the potency and combination of ingredients. Careful balance and thoughtful study to create an effective formula is a must when edging toward radical results.

Ingredients are ingredients, but how and when to use them is the key. You'll hear more about that as we move forward. Just as there is a formula for creating the strongest skincare that can also be used on sensitive skin, there is a powerful formula that can be used to create a meaningful and radical life. We will share that prescription formula with you.

For years we have worked with some of the most influential mentors, success coaches, and spiritual leaders in the world to discern that certain ingredients are always present when people are building success and living their dreams.

REVERSE ENGINEERING

From our perspective, the clearest path to accomplishing our goal was reverse engineering: Identify the problem and work backwards to create elixirs that could provide the solutions. Applying this concept to your life, we all have certain traits that support us and are part of our individual winning formulas. There are other traits that we carry that do not support us. So we may need to compensate, add a bit more to the formula, and be a bit more rigorous in the areas that are not our strengths. But if you identify the destination, know where you are and where you are going, you can work backwards to map out the journey to reach it.

Live "The Radical Yes"

	In Skincare	In Life
No excuses. No regrets.	✓	✓
Power and potency.	✓	✓
Honest and real.	✓	✓
Elegant and efficient.	✓	✓
We want it all.	✓	✓
We want it now.	✓	✓
More is better.	✓	✓
No time to waste.	✓	✓
Making a difference.	✓	✓

To better understand and appreciate the idea of a radical formula, let's take a look at a couple of women who have created their own prescription to living a radical life.

RADICAL thought

Changing your skin and your life requires the same core methodology. The key is that you must be radical in your approach.

Our dear friend Lavinia Errico, the founder of Equinox Health Clubs, shared the ingredients she used to create a radical life: "Courage, tenacity, and guts – these ingredients allowed me to understand that I am a strong person. The biggest thing is having the courage to figure out who you really are. Everything starts with you. What is your truth? Find strength and courage. Find autonomy. Just believe. Believe in the universe. Believe that everything will be fine no matter what the outcome looks like. Practice gratitude and

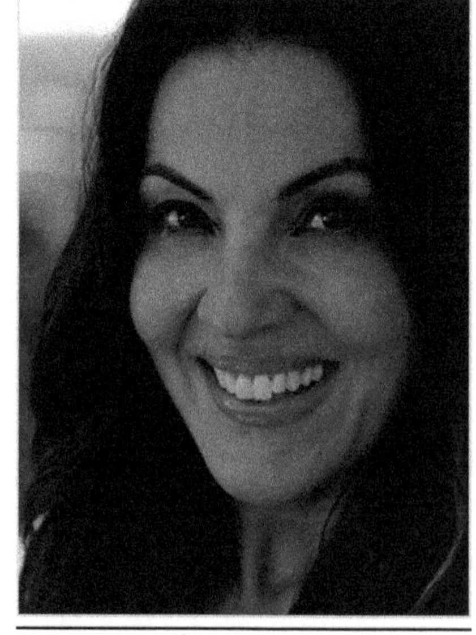

Equinox Founder Lavinia Errico

acceptance on a deep level. Feeling good comes from within. Take the journey of self-discovery." Recently Lavinia's husband developed cancer. As brutal as the diagnosis, treatments, and fear were, she refers to the process as a blessing that brought courage and honest sharing to the forefront. Lavinia uses even her greatest life challenges as fuel for her growth.

Tracey Woodward grew up with a drug-addicted mother who left Tracey to raise her little brother at the cost of a traditional education. Tracey would help with housekeeping jobs and do whatever it took to contribute to the family. At the age of fourteen, Tracey still could not read or write. But she would not let her lack of education get in the way of her dream and belief of future success. She simply would squeeze her size 5 $^{1}/_{2}$ foot into a size 3 shoe and attend an interview for a counter girl at Clinique. She got the job, and since that day has dominated in excellence in the field of beauty. From Clinique to Donna Karen, and now a strategic advisor to the mega-companies like M&S, Tracey still asserts that her core values allowed her to survive and thrive. She told us the radical ingredients she adds to her life are: "Honesty, compassion, balance, self-belief, and enthusiasm. Additionally, charm and good social skills are essential for success. People never remember what you say or do, but they always remember how you make them feel. So make them feel the best you possibly can, and in turn you will also feel good. Think about how you want to be treated, and understand that we are all mirrors of each other. To get it, you have to give it, so why wait to get it? Just give it to everybody until it comes back to you!"

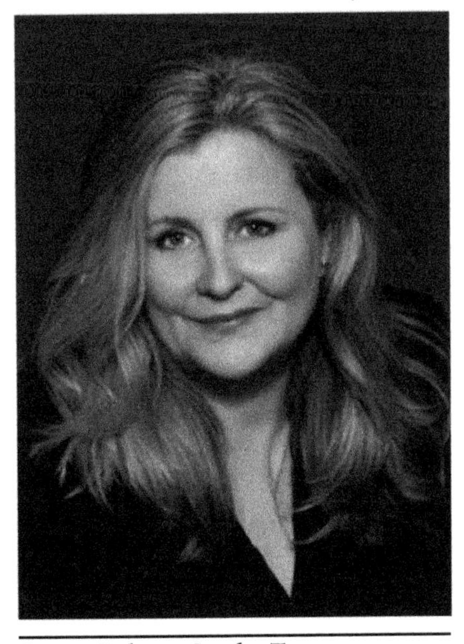

Beauty Industry Leader Tracey Woodward

She continues, "Goals are important for moving forward. We can always ask ourselves, 'What's next?' This will help keep us goal focused and will allow us to visualize a better life. Positive visualization is powerful. Remember, we can't change the past, so instead of dwelling, we need to move forward. Also, it helps to remember that we are all the same. If we can just talk openly and have no element of shame about who we are or where we come from or how we got here, it is very easy to move forward without the baggage. The only person holding you back is you. Whether you think you can or you can't, you are right. It is hard to go out and make opportunities, but you can if you choose to. You only have one life. This is it. So plan what you want to achieve and make the most of it."

Our friends above do a great job of sharing the radical ingredients they chose to mix together.

Remember, the process is grounded in finding the right mix and the right strength. With it, miracles can happen. Your radical life will be manifested. But it takes time. And effort. And tinkering. And the absolute desire to succeed. We all want a radical life. Our goal throughout this book is not only to give you a glimpse of what's possible, but also to show you how to turn that glimpse into a vision, and turn your dreams into achievable goals.

To that end, the next few chapters will break down what we view as the radical prescription you'll need to build a radical life that you love. When you incorporate these ingredients into a formula for your life, we are confident that you will begin to transform your life into an exciting and extensively radical one.

Chapter 3:
RADICAL PRESCRIPTION

An important starting point is to honestly take a look at where you are right now. You have to know where you are to know how to get where you are going.

What our two amazing friends and mentors above remind us is that you have to get honest with who and where you are *today* so you can figure out where you want to be *tomorrow*. Have gratitude and acceptance, and then embrace a new way of getting where you want to go.

We all experience life in a certain way. We do it in a radical way. For just a moment assume that you want more and that it is possible for you to have all that you want, but your way isn't getting you there. If you are not getting there your way, then why not try ours? Try getting radical in your approach. What do you have to lose?

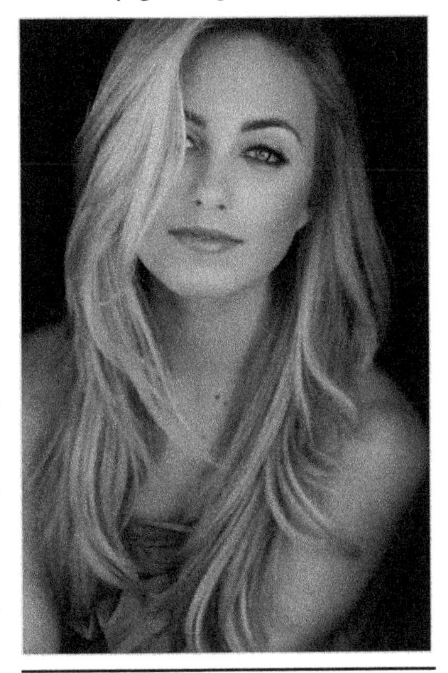

Miss Florida 2014, Tori Cowen

It was at an event honoring Radical Women who make a difference where we met Tori Cowen who, in 2014, was crowned Miss Florida. Tori is a real inspiration. During her tenure, she drove over 5000 miles per month, speaking to thousands about reaching their dreams. Her message is simple: no matter what walls are before you, getting radical in your viewpoint and your approach can take you there.

Tori shares, "As a woman, when I am faced with a challenge, the first step I take is changing my viewpoint. A challenge can look like an unmovable wall in front of your face. Yet, you will never know the benefits of what is behind that wall until it is removed. So I challenge you today to change your viewpoint. Imagine what it would look like if that wall were removed. Imagine how your life would look, how it would change, how it would evolve. What would it feel like if you overcame the challenge? Conquered the unconquerable? Then, write down the necessary steps it will take to overcome the challenge, with the benefits in mind."

Life can be a blur, but by being radical and thinking radical in the moment, so many doors will open that will create new roads and opportunities to be all that you can be. By being radical, you can have a life full of love, abundance, and ultimate fulfillment. Imagine what that would look and feel like for you.

Maintaining a radical lens to view the world has often supported and strengthened the fabric of our being; we constantly look for the golden opportunities to turn life into a wild and exciting ride. Buddha said, "Your purpose in life is to find your purpose and give your whole heart and soul to it."

With Radical, we did just that. And as we continued on our own journeys, and saw how these principles for success changed our lives, we felt compelled to share them with you. What good is an asset if you don't share it with others?

Building the Radical Skincare line from the bottom up took dedication, determination, and eventually a very specific prescription of ingredients that were tirelessly tested and retested. But simply launching this line and delivering life-changing skincare wasn't enough. We knew we also had the ability to deliver life-changing secrets and a philosophy that could change your life and reignite and brighten the light and passion behind your eyes.

At first we were intrigued, and then we became obsessed, with the relationship between our journey and your journey. We knew we could make a radical difference in your life because we made it in our own. And so was born our commitment to write this book.

We began identifying the *how* beneath our *what* that constantly led us to the door of opportunity. There simply had to be a way to apply our path for skincare transformation to the journey of life. We knew there was a clear-cut path and blueprint for living a radical life, and in the spirit of science (which we grew up with) a specific prescription that you can follow. That prescription started with identifying and understanding the essential ingredients we have always relied upon. We also determined that without a prescription or recipe, ingredients mean very little. It is the prescriptive recipe that takes the ingredients and gives them the life they need to truly gain enormous potential.

We began by asking questions like:

- *What are some of the key ingredients that the most successful and happy people we know, and have studied, attribute their success to?*
- *Are there consistent decisions and actions that support living a radical life?*
- *If so, how do they interact with one another to build a meaningful and exciting experience?*
- *And, much like our ingredients for Radical Skincare, can they be bottled up and offered for public consumption?*

Answering these questions took a lot of inner reflection and evaluation. But the result, much like our skincare line, is that there are very succinct and results-oriented ingredients that can lead to a potent yet accessible prescription for a radical life.

TURNING ABOUT-FACE

Radical Ingredients
Radical Ingredients include:
Authenticity
Balanced
Belief
Compassion
Courage
Goal-oriented
Integrity
Kindness
Passion
Resilience
Tenacity
Trust

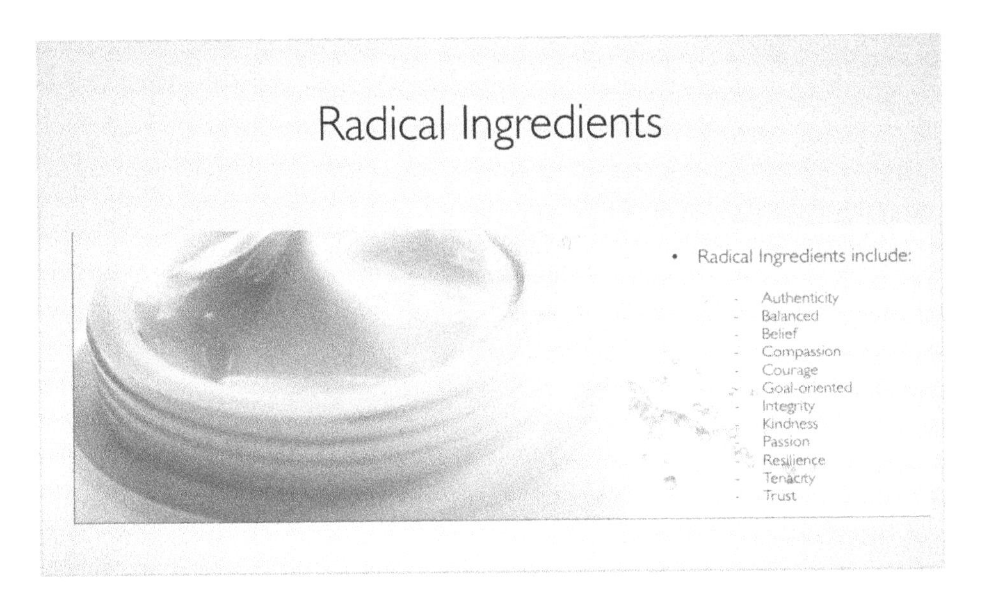

As women, as men, as people, we all have our own voyage and expedition, one that is unique to our experiences, our purpose, our passion, and our ultimate goals – and one that includes plenty of other people who came before us and after us, who were all willing to offer amazing feedback and support to help us reach our goals.

RADICAL thought | Surround yourself with people who believe in you and see your potential.

Thus, it is important to include the stories and advice these fantastic mentors offered. With their blessing, we will share their stories of how they built a radical life. And we are confident their outlook and stories will both inspire and serve as examples of exactly how you can build a meaningful, purpose-driven, and radical life, one day at a time. As Melanie Griffith, our close friend and famous actress, told us, "I define radical as truly living your life according to what you believe in. That's radical to me. And a lot of women don't realize that they can change their purview. They can change their perspective and live a radical life." For us, it is truly time to be the catalyst for that change.

But now is the time to turn the mirror onto you. Our goal is to serve you and your journey. You will learn about our lives and our experiences, which will act as the conduits through which we can together refocus your expedition and perhaps even completely change course. But we certainly recognize that, as women, we all carry a very special and unique right to passage.

RADICAL thought | Only when we turn about-face and go deeper than just the skin can we truly propose a very specific prescription for living a radical life.

This starts with nine very detailed and precise prescriptive statements that will act as the foundation for a radical life. After introducing them, we will break these important concepts down into approachable chunks so we can cement a foundation that you can build upon in your own unique way.

These include:

1. **Say the Radical Yes** – you never know when opportunity knocks.
2. **Recognize the potential in adversity** – it is always present.
3. **Understand your beliefs** – and rewrite them to serve you.
4. **Decisions lead to outcomes** – don't be afraid to make them.
5. **Identify your passion and purpose** – success and joy live there.
6. **Visualize the outcome you desire** – imagine big and see it with emotion.
7. **Set Goals** – write them down in the present tense, be specific, and read them often.
8. **Embrace opportunity** – it is there for you.
9. **Build a team that supports your dream** – they are your gift and you are theirs.
10. **Be a difference maker** – because you can.
11. **Welcome in Abundance** – consistently set goals, attract outcomes, and visualize dreams.

Above are nine simple yet powerful prescriptive steps. Each one played a significant role in our personal and professional journeys, and we are confident they will play a similar role for you. And each will be support for your growth, your transformation, and the changes you will welcome into your life to be more radical than you ever thought possible.

With that said, let's begin writing a radical prescription for living a life you love.

Chapter 4: RADICAL YES

So, where does our prescription begin? Well, unless you say *Radical Yes* to the journey ahead, you'll always find yourself stuck at the starting line, never even making your way out the gate. It takes a *Yes* to obtain great success.

We are all very familiar with that small and concise three-letter word, which is often perceived as more powerful than any other word in the English language.

Never forget it.

With it, you can open the floodgates of possibility.

It should always be on the tip of your tongue.

E.E. Cummings said, "It is the oldest living thing."

It breathes life into each of us.

And trust us when we say that with this word, you are armed with opportunity and always at the door of great success.

Just say it.

Yes.

Louder.

Yes.

You can never even imagine what can happen if you just say *yes.* And so, when it comes to radical ingredients, *yes* may be the first one we take off the shelves. One of the first ingredients we have identified in our quest to mix an elixir for a radical life is welcoming in a life filled with *Radical Yes* and never taking no for an answer.

Martin Luther King Jr. was told that equality was not possible.

Rosa Parks was informed she would have to give up her seat in the back of the bus to a white passenger.

Henry Ford was left penniless five times before he founded Ford Motor Company.

A newspaper editor fired Walt Disney because "he lacked imagination and had no good ideas."

Albert Einstein didn't speak until the age of four and didn't read until he turned seven.

Charles Darwin was often chastised by his father for being lazy and too dreamy.

Socrates was called "an immoral corrupter of youth" and sentenced to death.

Thomas Edison made one thousand unsuccessful attempts before inventing the light bulb.

Winston Churchill failed the sixth grade.

Jerry Seinfeld was booed off stage during his first standup performance.

Monet's style of painting was consistently rejected and mocked by the artistic elite.

Only after Isaac Newton failed at running his family farm was he sent away to Cambridge by an angry uncle.

Orville and Wilbur Wright built hundreds of failed prototypes before they created a plane that could get airborne and stay there.

Before becoming president, Abraham Lincoln was sent to war as a captain and was demoted to the lowest rank of private before he returned home.

At his first audition, Sidney Poitier was told by the casting director, "Why don't you stop wasting people's time and go out and become a dishwasher or something?"

And the list goes on. A *no* comes in many forms. Each of the renowned men and women above were told, "No, you cannot." But they did. And their gift to society is vast. The world would be a darker place without the people mentioned above (especially Edison). We all have similar journeys. You have to go through a lot of *no's* to get to even one *yes.*

Every single change the world sees starts with a Radical Yes!

Responding to the *no's* is just as important as accepting a *yes.* To make a difference, you need to have thick skin. You have to be willing to be so dedicated to your craft and your vision that you are unwilling to allow the opinions of others to sway you from your ultimate passion and purpose.

Radical means never taking no for an answer. The successful people we know who persevered in their goals and continued to move in the right direction, regardless of the number of *no's* they received on their journey, did it through accepting no other answer than a *yes.*

Remember, you may always be just one step away from reaching your goals.

We have the power to say *yes* to happiness and a multitude of opportunities that await us. We can decide to live the life of our dreams. However, to do so we also have to be willing to step outside of our comfort zone.

Radical Yes means embracing the things that both scare and excite you. It means pushing your own boundaries, breaking through your personal ceiling, and knowing that you can hit an achievable goal. Fear is a choice. Sure, there are times when there is reasonable and perceivable risk associated with choices. But fear is a state of mind, and ultimately it is your decision whether you should acknowledge your fear or simply ignore it.

In fact, your goals should be just a little uncomfortable, scary, and fear inducing. It keeps you honest. It tests your tenacity. It calls for grit. From the formulation of your life, the process of applying a new application, a new tool, or a new ingredient may slightly alter the path or direction of your journey. But saying *yes* to the opportunity, experience, or potential can often be the differentiator.

We call this the *Radical Yes.*

A *Radical Yes* encourages generosity and giving, and allows it to be part of your everyday life. Generosity doesn't have to be something so sacrificial that it's taxing or becomes a hardship. It's the nature of going beyond, in a moment, to make a difference because you can. It is about saying yes when others may just say no. It is about acting even when the action and its results are uncertain. Not because it's required or expected or necessarily needed, but the act itself makes someone's moment, day, or life better, which impacts the richness of your moment.

Life is a series of moments, and the more radical moments we string together, the more radical our life can be. It's the small moments of grace and proactive, positive creation that set the stage to make the change. Say the *Radical Yes* to generosity and know that it can be the smallest of things that make a radical difference in someone's day.

Of course, *yes* is a word that can also yield incredible power and momentum in the wrong direction if it is not used with judgment. So clearly we are not saying *yes* to things we intuitively know may destroy all that we intend on creating. Rather, say *yes* to new experiences, people, places, hobbies, etc., instead of "No, I am too busy, I can't... the kids... my husband, etc." You are embracing the freedom to say *yes* and knowing that the world will still be there when you return. In fact, the world will probably reward you when you say *yes.* And when you return you may do so with a renewed sense of richness, experience, energy, and vitality to share.

Liz: At twenty-five, I moved to Los Angeles. The move was not planned. I did not know anyone there. I didn't have much money and had no guarantee of success. It all started because I took a "buying trip" with a friend who owned a boutique. I always liked the idea of year-round sun and palm trees, and I had been to LA only once before at age eighteen. So seven years later I thought I would take another look at California from a different vantage point. I was a stockbroker in Virginia at the time, and my manager set me up with Cynthia, a successful female broker in Beverly Hills. She and I were comparing career notes and talking about our lives, our boyfriends, and all the things that were causing us untold pain, along with our desire to be, do, and have more.

At the end of lunch she said, "Come on, move out to California. We are going to be best friends." (And in fact, to this day, we are.)

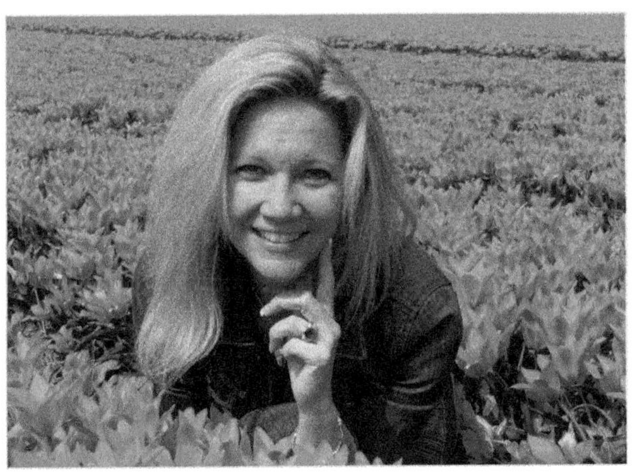

Longtime Friend Cynthia LaRoche

To most, including me, that sounded rather insane. My business was in Virginia, my family and friends were in Virginia, the home I had purchased was there, and I didn't have a lot of money. I was also in a destructive relationship that I seemed incapable of ending for good. So I thought, *maybe three thousand miles of distance will fix it!* I said *yes* and proceeded to call all of my friends and clients to inform them of my decision to move to LA before I changed my mind. I wanted to put enough pressure on myself to stick to this decision and embrace this new adventure. It would be too easy to go home, get back into my routine, think of all the reasons why I shouldn't take a risk, or play it safe and succumb to the fears that seemed more practical and legitimate than following a hunch, radical intuition, and a dream.

So there it was – the little *yes* that totally changed my life. Within two weeks I moved to Beverly Hills, California, with my clothes and my car. I moved into a hotel that I got a discount on since my brother worked for the company, and I began a new life.

As I looked around my room with rolling clothing racks stacked two deep, I wondered what I was thinking. But I had a vision. And the possibilities that lay ahead simply had to be better than what lay behind me. I knew who I was and what I had in Virginia. I knew the life path that I was inching down, and it was not reflective of my dream. Of something bigger. Of me being more and taking risks and stretching. So I took a deep breath and kept my sights focused on my dream and vision of possibility.

Within three years I had built a successful business and was on my way to managing half a billion dollars. I had traveled the world, and I would soon meet my husband. All of this became a reality because of a chance meeting, saying yes to a dream, and taking a risk.

A goal that doesn't reflect extreme desire has no real excitement, emotion, or energy behind it. The passionate feeling of engagement and desire is an ingredient that will drive a person to do what it takes, and also put the universe in action to deliver your heart's desire. People are afraid to fail, so the fear of wanting something and not having it happen can be paralyzing. Part of being radical is to suspend judgment and give yourself the generous gift of believing and owning a desire even if you don't know how it will occur. And that starts with embracing the opportunity to say *yes.* The best news is that these occasions present themselves almost every day. Life presents us with a myriad of opportunities to which we can respond with a *Radical Yes!*

A life centered on *Radical Yes* is one where a father dresses up to have a tea party with his daughter, the "princess;" it is a dissatisfied employee quitting her job to follow her lifelong dream of starting a non-profit; a stay-at-home mother opening an online cupcake company to fill her downtime; an unhappy wife taking a trip out of the country on her own to find meaning in her life; a young man converting a room in his apartment into an art studio so he can paint after work. But, most importantly, it is saying *yes* when you were once inclined to say no.

Remember, it was the *yeses* of Martin Luther King Jr., of Walt Disney, of Henry Ford, of Rosa Parks, of Albert Einstein, and of so many more great thinkers and visionaries that literally changed the world. They each maintained their respective dreams and relied on their own unique sets of ingredients to reach their goals and fulfill their destinies. They were radical. And they each whispered the word *yes* over and over again while every other person around them was yelling *no.* It was that *Radical Yes* that led the way and maintained the light needed to guide them through the darkness of a world filled with *no's.*

When confronted with a YES or NO decision, always remember that:

We may always be just one step away from reaching our goals, so the more we say "Yes," the more opportunities that are before us to uncover and discover.

Radical Yes means embracing the things that both scare and excite you.

Say *Radical Yes* to generosity, fun, love, sharing, doing, and laughing; it is in giving and receiving that our lives transform.

Most importantly, it is saying *Yes* when you were once inclined to say no.

Get Radical. Say Yes to life.

The following is a framed quote that hangs on Cynthia's wall as a reminder to her to say "Yes" to life.

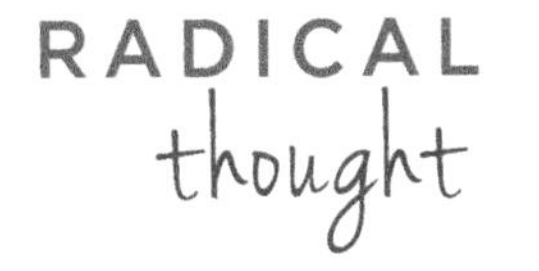

The following is a framed quote that hangs on the wall of Cynthia's bathroom as a reminder to her.

To laugh is to risk appearing the fool.

To weep is to risk appearing sentimental.

To reach out for another is to risk involvement.

To risk feelings is to risk exposing your true self.

To place your ideas, your dream, before a crowd is to risk their loss.

To love is to risk not being loved in return. To live is to risk dying.

To hope is to risk failure.

But risks must be taken,

Because the greatest hazard in life is to risk nothing and do nothing.

You dull your spirit.

You may avoid suffering and sorrow,

But you cannot learn, feel, change, grow and live.

Chained by your attitude, you are a slave.

You have forfeited your freedom.

Only if you risk are you free.

Radical Recap:

When confronted with a YES or NO decision, always remember that:

1. We may always be just one step away from reaching our goals, so the more we say "Yes," the more opportunities that are before us to uncover and discover.
2. Radical Yes means embracing the things that both scare and excite you.
3. Say Radical Yes to generosity, fun, love, sharing, doing, and laughing; it is in giving and receiving that our lives transform.
4. Most importantly, it is saying Yes when you were once inclined to say no.
5. Get Radical. Say Yes to life.

I believe in pink.
I believe that
laughing is the best
calorie-burner.
I believe in kissing,
kissing a lot.
—Audrey Hepburn

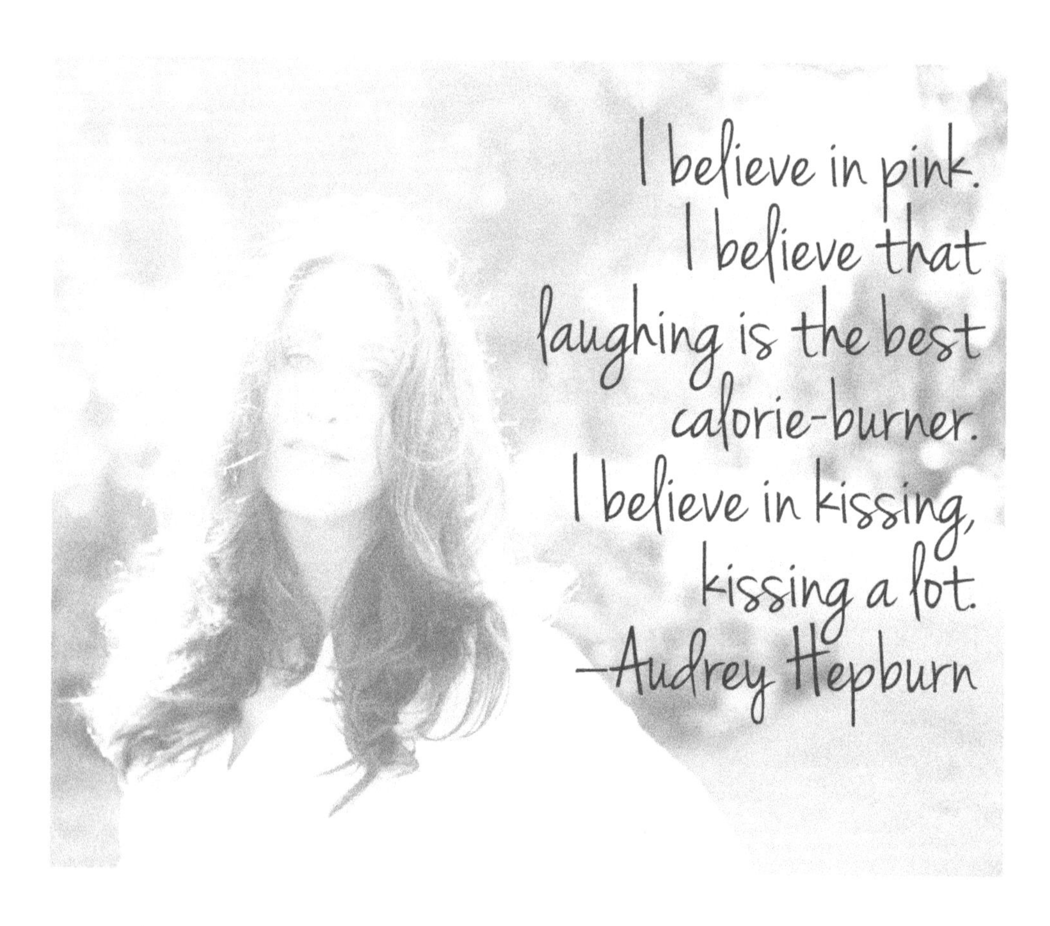

Chapter 5:
RADICAL ADVERSITY

So that brings us to our next ingredient for creating a radical prescription for life. Adversity isn't always the easiest pill to swallow, and it can certainly leave a bad taste in your mouth. But the truth of the matter is that the greatest opportunities are often the ones forged from adversity.

Opportunity.

Napoleon Hill told us, "Your big opportunity may be right where you are now."

You never know…

Thomas Edison reminded us that most people miss opportunity because "It is dressed in overalls and looks like work."

No one said it would be easy.

But maybe it was Winston Churchill who said it best when he stated, "An optimist sees the opportunity in every difficulty."

Adversity.

Welcome adversity with open arms.

Zig Ziglar reminds us, "Sometimes adversity is what you need to face in order to become successful."

View it as an obstacle on your journey to success.

Malcolm X said, "There is nothing better than adversity. Every defeat, every heartbreak, every loss contains its own seed, its own lesson on how to improve your performance the next time."

Plant the seeds and nurture them.

Tracey Woodward says, "Look for the good in every incident. When it's bad, it never stays the same and when it's good, it never stays the same. The point is that everything changes."

In fact, the altitude of success is often born out of the depths of failure.

We have always felt that radical living calls for a radical attitude. Part of that attitude, and an important ingredient to building a fulfilling and radical life, is understanding that there is a healthy relationship between opportunity and adversity. In fact, most of the time you cannot have one without the other. Yin to the yang.

TURN ADVERSITY INTO OPPORTUNITY

We have had many challenges over the years, many of which have forced us to figure out a way to go over it, around it, or under it. Simply put, we had to find a better way. They say what doesn't kill you makes you stronger. We actually hate that line, because we tend to hear it when we feel like we are crumpled over on our knees at a painful place in life.

Collectively, we've had numerous challenges and adversities on our life journey. We watched our father suffer from MS, which not only destroyed him physically but also accosted the family dynamic as we fought to survive it. Abusive relationships. Divorce. Our mother breaking under stress and anxiety and eventually developing dementia. And the list goes on. What is important about this litany of adversities is how you grow from it all and, after applying radical principles, how you continue to move in the direction of your dreams.

Liz: A big moment of adversity for me occurred after I had funded a diet company in my venture capital days and put my money, investor's money and my friend's money into the company. My sister, who was working there, called me one day and said, "Liz, the president of the company has a drug problem, my paycheck bounced, and I think he has been taking the money that you, your friends and clients invested."

For me it was a disaster. I had so much at stake. I felt depressed, vulnerable and like a failure. It can happen to any of us at any point in time. I was in LA; I had just left a four-year relationship, breaking off our engagement. I had left the home I was living in with him (in which I had invested most of my savings in home improvement, thinking we were forever). On top of it, I didn't document my investment and had no recourse. So there I sat, in my newly rented house that Rachel and I referred to as "the crib," where we would start again. I sat at the bottom of the stairs, staring out at the City of Angels in tears, wondering how I was ever going to get our money out of this company and how I would build my financial life yet again.

They say it is darkest before the dawn. Well, it felt pretty dark. So I reached out for help. I called some friends in the finance business and asked if they knew of a lawyer that was tough who would help me out of this mess. And, by the way, I told them, "I don't have any money for a retainer." All three friends recommended the same lawyer and called him and requested that he take my call. He did. He took my case on a contingency basis. After over a year of litigation hell, he won my money and my friend's money back with interest. He actually got the judge to award me the entire company and got rid of the drug-addicted owner. And the craziest part to the story is... I married that same lawyer!

I went from leaving a relationship, to losing money and feeling a sense of despair, to getting the money back, owning a new wellness and weight-loss company, working with my sister in this new industry (which launched our careers in health and wellness), to marrying the lawyer who took my case on contingency. Just one example of adversity to opportunity.

PURPOSE OVERRIDES ADVERSITY

It is amazing how a sense of purpose can light a fire in your soul and propel you to overcome seemingly impossible situations. It can make you suddenly feel alive when you have felt like you were on automatic.

Our good friend Baroness Patricia Scotland of Asthal is a radical example of someone who turns adversity into opportunity. In 1991 she became the first black woman ever to be appointed as Queen's Counsel, in 1997 she became life member of the House of Lords, and in 2007 she went on to become the first female attorney general. Born in the Commonwealth of Dominica as the tenth child of twelve, her life was a pursuit of radical proportions from an early age. Throughout her remarkable career she has made real inroads toward eliminating domestic violence: her programs

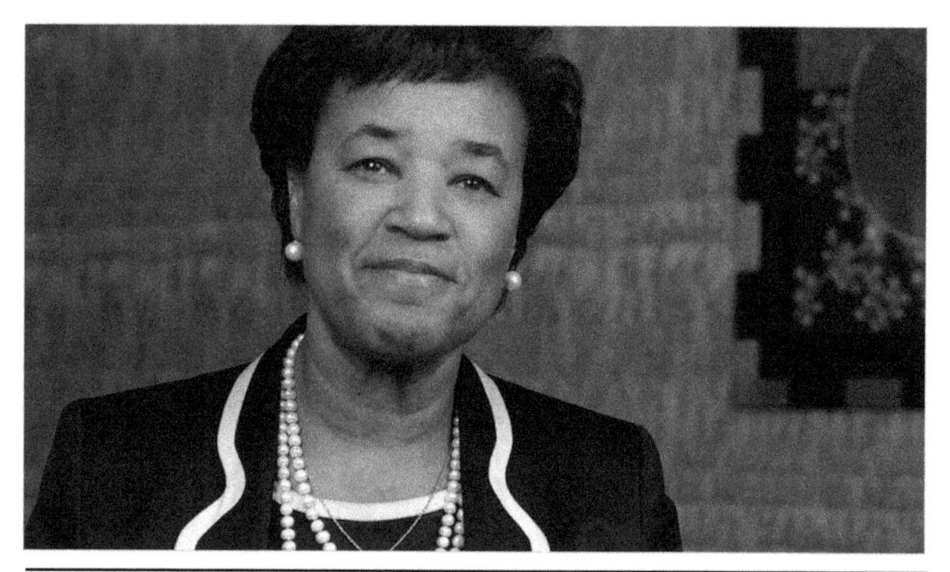

Baroness Patricia Scotland, past Attorney General for England and Wales and the first woman in 700 years to be in the House of Lords.

reduced the number of reported incidents in the UK by 64 percent. She spoke with us about the phenomenal perseverance and passion that make her a radical change maker while sharing the keys to creating change and success against all odds.

For more about Baroness Patricia Scotland's story visit her Living Portrait on the Radical Living section of our website *www.radicalskincare.com/living.*

Radical Living section of our website.

"I feel very blessed because both of my parents led us to believe that every single person under God's heaven is given a talent, and it is our job to find that talent, to hone it, and then use it for the benefit of other people," Baroness Scotland told us. "I became the only woman in over seven hundred years to be appointed as Her Majesty's Attorney General. I remember thinking, *Everyone told me that I couldn't make it because I didn't have the right background, I didn't have the right skin color, and I wasn't a man* – I mean, I was just all wrong and I was never going to succeed. I think one of the most important things is not to accept things as they are, especially if they could be better. If you want to make a radical difference, you have to identify where change needs to happen."

Baroness Patricia identified an opportunity to transform adversity into opportunity when she coordinated a countrywide effort to eliminate domestic violence. She explains:

"One in three women in our world suffers from domestic violence. In our country, England, it is one in four. Domestic violence affects about 750,000 children per year, and I was told, 'you can't change that.' But I believed we could make a radical difference and we could change that, if only we joined together. We reduced domestic violence by 64 percent and we saved $7.1 billion a year in economic cost. And we did that by working together and being willing to be radical in the way we thought about delivering change. Don't ever be afraid of failing. Be terrified of not trying because if you don't try, you'll never know, and I've always found that the real radical thing to do is to say, 'I am walking, even if I walk on my own, but will you walk with me?' If we could get peace in the home, I think we'd have peace in the world."

RADICAL *thought*

"Don't ever be afraid of failing.
Be terrified of not trying."
– Baroness Patricia Scotland

Her radical perseverance has had an enormously positive impact on her country and the lives of countless individuals. She did not let adversity or challenges deter her from her goals or purpose to help others.

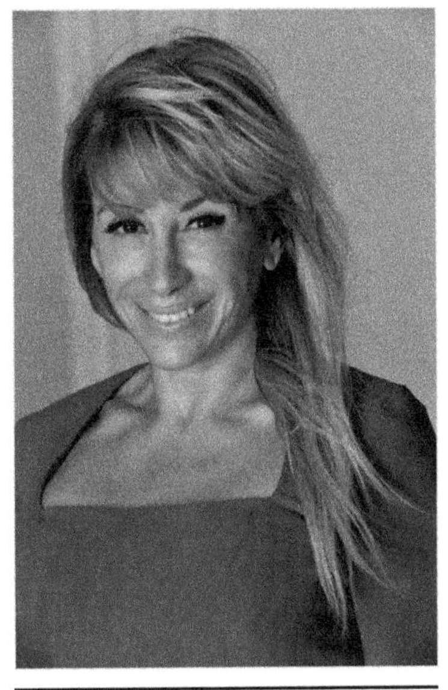

Princess Sophie Audouin-Mamikonian author of the best selling Tara Duncan book series

Is there a time when someone has told you that what you desire is not possible or that you don't have the background, money, experience, education, age, or whatever else you need to succeed? Maybe it wasn't someone else who told you this; maybe it was you that told yourself such a story, and that inner-doubt kept you from pursuing your dreams.

Our friend Princess Sophie Audouin-Mamikonian author of the best selling Tara Duncan book series which has sold over 11 million copies to date, shares the adversity she faced in launching this iconic book collection.

"I was 25 years old when I began to write Tara Duncan. For seventeen years I sent the book to publisher after publisher, and each time they said 'no'. I received over 300 letters of refusal saying, 'No we don't want your book, no we don't like your book.' Can you imagine the frustration? You know that you have a good story; you know that you have a good book. So I just I kept going. I kept sending the book to other publishers, year after year after year and finally I got a yes and 11 million books later I have touched and inspired millions of young girls. Don't ever give up. Never. Go after your dream."

Each and every challenge presents an exciting occasion to rise to the top and find a solution, but first you have to go deep. You cannot let the wave of adversity stop you. Imagine you are in a sea full of waves knocking you around. You come up against some huge waves, a huge set, and you're swimming and trying to stay on top but you can barely respond or catch your breath. The only way to create true clarity is to take a deep breath and dive deep – deep, deep down beneath all the turmoil. In that quiet, in that depth, you will find the capability to look above you at the turmoil instead of being within it. It is there that you will get your strength to see clearly and carry on.

Our good friend Lavinia Errico shared her views on adversity. She says, "You've got to make life happen. You have to be the warrior. Be willing to take a risk and have the courage to fail. Failing is a great thing because it means you are doing something. It takes a lot of courage to do that. It takes so much courage to be like, 'Alright, I am gonna look failure right in the eye, and I am still moving forward.' You can't have a breakthrough without a breakdown. Be okay with it and accept it. Now is not the time to run away from it. Another way of looking at it is that you have to have a crisis to have a healing. If you avoid the crisis, you avoid the healing."

When we avoid our problems, we don't move forward. We must have the courage to look adversity in the eye and face failure. When we do this, we find a way toward success.

Our Uncle Ted Edlich is the author of *Navigating the Rapids of Non-Profit Leadership* and was the president and CEO of Total Action Against Poverty. TAP is the largest private non-profit human development and community development organization in Southwest Virginia, serving urban, suburban, and rural communities in the area. TAP projects address the issues of housing, healthcare, education, economic development, criminal justice, transportation, and energy conservation.

Uncle Ted is committed to bringing the community together to overcome stereotypes and create institutional change that results in equal opportunity for all regardless of race, ethnic background, sex, and family economic status. For us growing up, Uncle Ted was the giant crab that would chase us around the living room and tickle us. For our Dad, Ted was the older brother – the shining light that protected Dad and pushed him to dive into school and athletics to escape his volatile home situation. Like Uncle Ted worked to save our Dad, he took those same protective and big brotherly qualities and dedicated his life to serving underprivileged communities. Uncle Ted's radical view on attacking impoverished communities and the adversity they face can be applied to our lives as well.

He told us, "From the beginning, I think one of the most radical things about our approach was likely the simplest part of it. The secret lay in asking the question and listening. Our goal was to actually listen to low-income families themselves to get their take on what their problems or adversity looked like. In rural communities in Southwest Virginia, we were involved in a project where we sent outreach workers and community organizers to ask people: 'What's your biggest problem?' The consistent response was that they did not have any drinking water or outdoor plumbing. They had to either bail it out of a creek, borrow it from a neighbor, or buy it from the store. It was the act of going out to those folks and asking a simple question and listening to their answer that allowed TAP to implement a radical response to overcome adversity. We developed a water development program for them that eventually went national. *It was inquiring into their adversity that started radical change across the country.*"

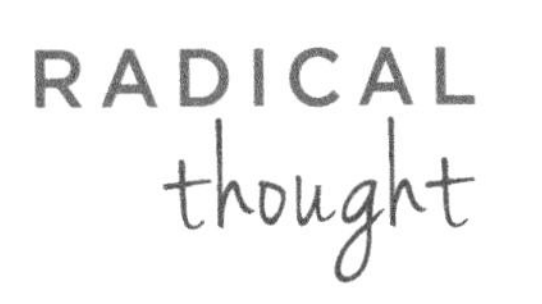

Find your radical solution by embracing opportunity through understanding your adversity. What is your challenge? What do you perceive as your adversity? What is your purpose?

Rachel: I believe this sense of purpose-driven energy is a key o handling challenging places in life. In fact, I can now say that I don't overcome a challenge, I take on a challenge. Challenge? Okay. Bring it on. What'd ya got? Throw it at me. I can do it. So I don't think of it as having to overcome challenges because that makes me feel like a victim. Instead, I kind of maneuver around and take a different approach and come at it a different way. I take on, and effectively handle, challenges every single day.

As Albert Einstein says, *"In the middle of difficulty lies opportunity."*

As we put one foot in front of the other and realized that our journey was not just skin-deep, our inner drive and outward purpose began to brighten the lives of those around us. We made a difference. We turned our challenge into an opportunity to serve others.

RESILIENCE IS RADICAL

The name Melanie Griffith is synonymous with Hollywood royalty. Melanie was nominated for an Academy Award and won a Golden Globe for her outstanding performance in *Working Girl,* a film that had a cultural empowerment impact on working women around the world. We met Melanie eighteen years ago through a fitness trainer friend of ours. As women on a personal and purposeful journey, we instantly connected and authentically shared our life challenges with one another.

"I am very resilient: as a woman, as a mother, as a person," Melanie said. "Sobriety was the biggest challenge for me. That was a huge hurdle for me to cross. I think we all have to make a choice in life: Are you a resilient person? Do you want to be the person who falls down but gets back up and keeps going? Or do you want to be the person who falls down and becomes the victim? I don't believe in self-wallowing. And I have done that at points in my life and really felt sorry for myself. You're either self-aware or you're self-conscious. I don't want to be self-conscious. I want to be quietly self-aware and self-possessed and be giving. The more you help other people, the more the world will give you back. Somehow things will magically open up for you and you'll create an amazing life."

Melanie has always been one to lead with love and share her struggles honestly in hopes that her journey empowers another. She continues to commit to taking adversity head on. She has been sober for years now; her youngest is off to college, and she has just consummated her divorce and has sold and moved out of the place that she called home for close to twenty years. Any one of these things would be considered a lot to deal with. As we were catching up, she said, " Going through this stuff is hard. Recreating your world is not easy. But I feel like I am a caterpillar that is molting and releasing a lot of 'stuff' that just wasn't working. I am now free to be a new and better me and take one day at a time."

As you are looking at challenges that are before you, know that a new and better you awaits as you shed your skin of yesterday and embrace what's possible.

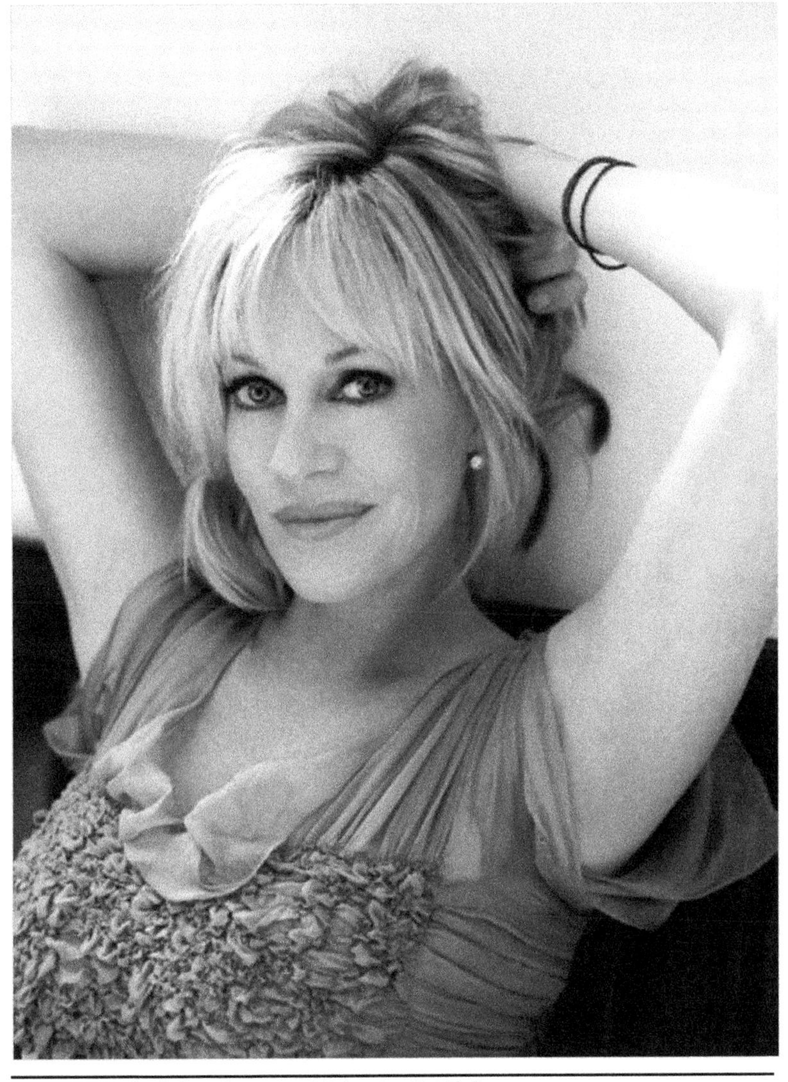

Actress and philanthropist Melanie Griffith

For more about Melanie Griffith's story visit her Living Portrait on the Radical Living section of our website www.radicalskincare.com/living.

RADICAL *thought* | Adversity builds strength and character. Overcoming adversity is radical.

So there is the second ingredient to living a radical life: finding radical opportunity through adversity. It is not always easy. Sometimes it is pretty difficult. Beauty and magic will become visible when you face adversity and persevere against the odds. You can achieve great things when you believe in yourself and all that life has to offer.

GOING ABOVE AND BEYOND YOUR ADVERSITY

Remember, the heat of adversity burns the blueprint of opportunity into your life. The more adversity you experience and then overcome, the stronger you will be and the more you will have to share with others to inspire them to be radical.

RADICAL *thought* | Take every failure as an opportunity to be better. Half the battle is recognizing it in the moment!

Liz: Personally, nothing has taught me more than the purpose-driven fortitude of my own father. Dad, Dr. Richard F. Edlich, went on to become one of the most awarded reconstructive surgeons and authors in medicine today all in the face of his adversity. He had the option to make millions of dollars in private practice, but instead he chose to remain on staff in esteemed universities so his findings and research could forward medicine and make a difference in the world. His career is replete with contributions, from the development of Steri-Strips, which he GAVE to 3M, to founding the Burn Unit at the University of Virginia, to revolutionizing emergency medical services in our country, as we know it. He won many seemingly impossible battles in medicine, but none were as breathtaking as the fact that most of his contributions in the last twenty-five years were from a wheelchair.

Through his assistants and caregivers, Dad dictated, did research, worked with medical students, petitioned the FDA on the dangers of latex powdered gloves, and published numerous peer-reviewed articles annually. He did all of this using his voice and his unwavering focus and determination to make a difference.

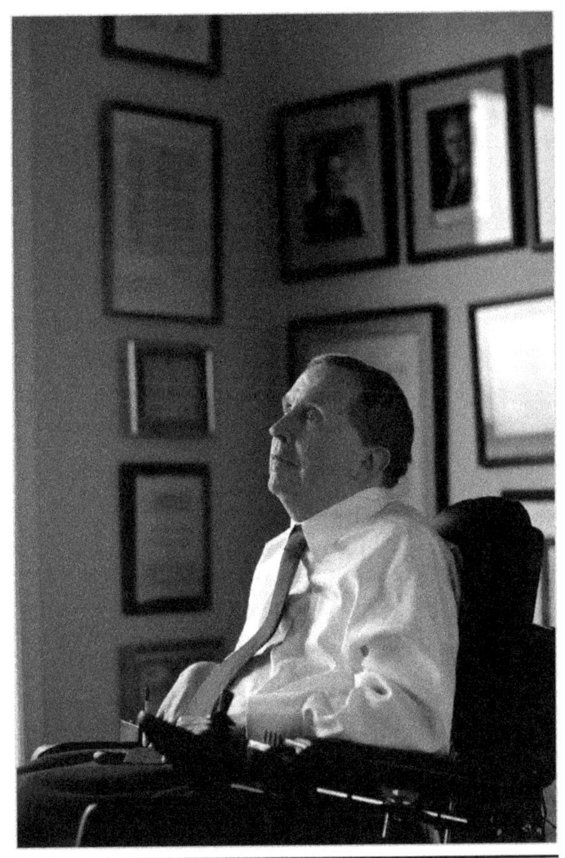

Dr. Richard F. Edlich, MD, PHD and Distinguished Professor of Plastic Surgery and Professor of Biomedical Engineering: Photo courtesy of Portland Oregon Photographer Craig Mitchelldyer www.craigmitchelldyer.com

His purpose to make a difference, right the wrong, and encourage others to reach their dreams allowed him to overcome his physical challenges. It is the passion for something greater than his own life that drove him and forged his missions. There is no doubt in my mind that growing up with him as our Dad and experiencing such purpose and determination has fueled my own drive as well as my sister's. More importantly, I believe that purpose fuels passion and desire, whether it is the drive to love and support a child, rid the world of disease, or create a fun environment for learning – the examples are endless. I believe it's a sense of purpose that drives the ordinary to do the extraordinary that makes the difference.

Ask yourself questions like:

- What lights me up? No matter how big or small it may be. Make a list.
- When is it that I feel alive?
- When do I lose track of time because I am so into the moment?
- What are the challenges before me?

- Am I looking my challenges in the eye and moving towards them?
- If I am not taking action, why not? List the reasons.
- How would I feel if I worked past the challenge before me?
- What could be possible if I just took a chance?
- What will it cost me if I do nothing?
- How does that make me feel?

At this point in our lives, Radical Skincare and making a radical difference in the lives of others gives us purpose and passion. Being inspired to be there for others, doing something outside of our boundaries, and embracing our mission offers our lives passion.

What breathes passion into you?

Whatever it is, use it as a cure for a case of adversity. Sometimes life will smack you right in the face. Sometimes it will feel like a jab, other times an uppercut to the chin. But how you respond to that big hit, or series of small jabs, will dictate whether or not you make it to the bell. Passion and purpose protect you from getting railroaded by adversity. Recognize that adversity is part of growth, part of the journey, and part of life. And how you handle it is what fuels your success.

Radical Recap:

When confronted with Radical Adversity, always remember that:

1. Each and every challenge presents an exciting occasion to rise to the top and find a solution, but first you have to go deep within yourself.
2. Ask questions and listen to yourself and others. What is at the core of the obstacle?
3. Reach out and ask for help.
4. Failure is an illusion and is just one step closer to obtaining what you want. Don't let the fear of failure stop you.
5. Let what you want be bigger than you and focus on that rather than the adversity at hand.
6. Beyond adversity awaits opportunity.
7. Nothing stays the same. Things are always changing.
8. Passion and purpose help drive action.

Chapter 6:
RADICAL DECISION MAKING

Decisions present a wonderful opportunity to embrace momentum and change. Some decisions will be great. Others are not so great. But the beauty is that you can decide again and grow from the learning. Refine and align your decisions with your goals, purpose, and passion to create real results and new experiences.

Yes or no, today or tomorrow, this way or that way, my way or your way, the current path or a different path? All of these decisions lead to unknown territory, uncertain results. Fear and trepidation can live in the moments before we make a decision. Excitement and expectations can live in those same moments. Regardless, decisions shape where we end up in our world.

Decision makers are truly difference makers.

Doctors have saved lives with decisions, juries have let innocent men go free, and our founders laid the foundation for our rights, liberties, and freedom of speech through the ones they wrote down on a little document in 1789, known as the "Bill of Rights."

Decisions.

For each of us, decisions are the true game-changers. They often define who we are and outline the parameters through which we live our lives. Make good ones and the sky is the limit.

But to build a radical life, the most important thing is to be the one to make decisions. Good, bad, or indifferent, be a decision-maker. Theodore Roosevelt said, "In any moment of decision, the best thing you can do is the right thing, the next best thing is the wrong thing, and the worst thing you can do is nothing."

So how can you make better decisions?

First of all, you have to be an independent thinker. In other words, you cannot be concerned with the opinions of other people. If you're concerned with the opinions of other people, you're never going to have an opinion of your own. That's very important to understand.

You have to be courageous. You know, Napoleon Hill said the majority of people who fail are generally influenced by the opinions of others. They permit the newspapers and the gossiping neighbors to do their thinking for them. Opinions are the cheapest commodity on earth. Everyone has a block of opinions ready to be wished upon anyone who will accept them. If you're going to be thwarted by the opinions of others, when you reach decisions they are not going to feel like they are truly yours.

Decisions are the basis of our lives. Big or small, the decisions we make shape our destiny. It all comes down to a series of different decisions you make. Good decisions, bad decisions, right decisions, wrong decisions. It's not all about the big decision, right? It's not all about that monumental, catastrophic, groundbreaking, earth-shattering decision you make or didn't make. It oftentimes can be a series of really small decisions that either serve as steps on a ladder to get you to the top, or create cracks in the foundation.

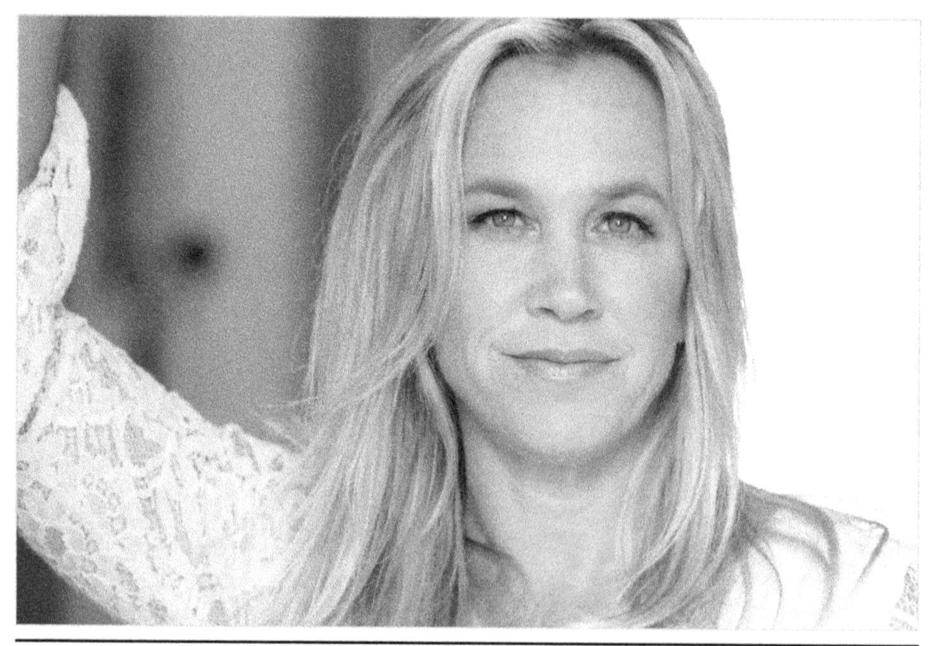

Rachel Edlich and her clear skin

Living a radical life is not always about the results of the decision. In fact, it is just the opposite. Living a radical life is about making the decision. Right, wrong, or indifferent, a radical life calls for you to weigh the outcomes and choose door number one or door number two. Remember, "If you stand in the middle of the road, you get hit by traffic going both ways." Indecision is a dangerous decision. So start by making a decision. Making decisions is one of the most important things you can do.

Every decision results in one of two outcomes: a good one or an adverse one. A good decision creates positive results in your life. An adverse decision offers the opportunity to learn from your mistakes. Either way, the result of your decision should be a welcomed one. It is indecision that can really hurt.

Through a radical lens, indecision is nonexistent. Indecision – saying I don't know, I can't decide – is actually making a decision. It's already decided. At times, remaining in a state of indecision falsely comforts us. But you actually make a decision by not making a decision at all.

Consider an example as easy as trying to decide if you should go to the gym. You tell yourself you are tired, hungry, and really not in the mood. So you are not ready to make a decision to go. Be clear: You have made a decision not to go to the gym at that time. Taking a job change or leaving a relationship that no longer serves you – In both cases you may say that you are not ready to make a decision to leave. But in both cases you MADE a decision. The decision was to stay at that moment. So empower yourself and say, "I am deciding to stay today." Own that decision until you are ready to choose differently.

RADICAL *thought* | When living a radical life, indecision is not your friend!

Now, we are not saying that you should do something you're not ready to do. There's a gestation period for everything in life. But it is a fallacy to live with false hope that indecision is a state that exists, because you choose something in every moment. Every moment is your choice. Indecision is a powerless state. You will find more opportunity and results the minute you shift your view to understand that in every single moment you choose – you choose to do something or not to do something. You choose to say something or not to say something. You choose to act or not to act. Those choices are what define and design the life you are living.

Rachel: We choose our day. We choose our conversations. Everything is a choice. We're making them all the time. That is a powerful place in which to live. And it is a fortunate one. We can all make choices. You learn from those choices that might not have worked out the way you planned, but at least you're moving forward. One way or another, you're doing something. Get in the game. The only way to win is to play. I have a strong moral compass that I operate from in all aspects of my life. This is the lens I look through when making decisions. Calibrate your own moral compass and use it to guide you when making decisions.

Liz: Go down swinging. Don't sit there and watch the ball. You're in the game of life. We always tell people to never just sit in the stands. Visually, indecision is sitting in the stands while everyone else is on the field and playing the game. Get out of the bleachers, and get down on the field and play. Remember, sitting in those rickety bleachers is a decision that ultimately will create your reality.

At the end of the day, decision is a sense of ownership. It is fundamentally fueled by the belief that you have complete and total control over your life. The most successful people make the most intentional decisions and the most mistakes. However, many feel that not making a decision is safer than making the wrong one. The consequences of doing nothing are substantial. Maimonides said, "The risk of a wrong decision is preferable to the terror of indecision." Keep putting one foot in front of the other; stay in constant movement with a refusal to remain stagnant and grow stale. Decision is the lubricant for growth. It allows you to usher in new opportunities and do away with old ones. With it, we evolve. Without it, we wither.

One of the biggest challenges with decisions is not just making a mistake, but that hard work or commitment may follow.

Rachel: I love it when I make a decision, and I love commitment. Get me committed because then I have something to hold on to. Going through my divorce and all the different things that happened was quite a challenge. Making those types of tough decisions is brutal. How I handled those moments was with the knowledge that there is something more, that there is something greater, that there is something better, and that this is all part of a big plan. It's unfolding perfectly. I say that to myself all the time when I'm feeling like I'm in a moment where I'm struggling with making a decision. Everything is unfolding perfectly just the way it's supposed to. I choose to believe that it's all working out in a perfect plan.

On a lighter note, some decisions are not as dramatic as divorce or a job change, yet they are decisions that build character. I made a decision to do a triathlon. Running and biking is not a problem for me. Being an athlete, I pretty much have confidence to see my way through. Give me a bike and I can ride. Throw me out there with running shoes and I can run. Swimming, however, is a different deal because I really have to work at it; I have to practice swimming. Swimming is not something where you jump in the water and you swim a mile. It just doesn't seem to work that way. Your breathing changes and you are trying to pace yourself, and it just seems unnatural and pushes you to your limits.

So for my first Sprint Triathlon, I had to prepare to swim a half-mile. I thought I would be ready if I swam every other day for half a mile in the pool. Well, not quite. The day of the race I jumped into the freezing ocean with a Tri-Suit on for the very first time and realized quickly that it wasn't that easy, as the hundreds of people were splashing and bumping into me trying to get their rhythm and space to swim. My heart rate was increasing, my breathing was out of sync, and panic started to set in. I immediately thought, *am I going to make it through this swim?* I was like, wow, I need to make a decision fast on how to get through this. I need a goal.

In triathlons – bike, run, and swim competitions – they have long boards all around the sides of the ocean swim, so if you are tired you can go and rest if you need to. My decision was not to touch one darn board! That was my goal. I'm swimming to swim, not to hold on. Staring at each board, I said to myself, *do not touch the board, do not touch the board.* I did it! I came out of the water and onto the bike and off to the run. I finished the race in the top ten for my age group. I was in shock considering that I thought I wouldn't complete it the moment I started swimming. How quickly that one decision helped me succeed. It was the baby steps in the moment and the confidence that I needed to keep going and take on the next challenge.

We make big decisions (and small ones) to grow and evolve. This behavior involves a daily commitment and a regular decision in each moment to keep going. To keep focused on a talk track that supports your desired goal. Make the decision on a moment-by-moment basis to have what you want. When you make a mistake or stall for a day or a short period of time, don't be discouraged because the next moment, the next hour, and the next day provides a new moment for you to make a different decision, one that brings you closer to your path.

For us, radical decisions means making decisions to create real results. Results are the target. That is why we do what we do. Whether it be results in the form of building a skincare line to solve our personal skin issues, or the results of creating a beautiful family, or starting a new business, or working to improve the quality of your life, it takes decisions to accomplish any and all of these.

Decisions are literally the lubricant for growth. Without them, you'll remain stagnant.

Thus, we are firm that the third ingredient to create a radical life is implementing a life filled with radical decisions. They don't have to be big, in fact they are mostly small, but they have to be made. One way or another, decisions will move you somewhere somehow.

To work towards making better decisions:

1. *Make a list of decisions that you have been putting off or are afraid to make.*
2. *Ask yourself: What am I gaining or losing by staying in the current state?*
3. *Ask yourself: What am I most afraid about when making a decision?*
4. *List decisions that you have made and how you have learned from them.*
5. *Ask yourself: What decisions must I make to move in the direction of my dreams?*
6. *Remember those times when you made decisions that changed your life for the better.*

Tori Cowen shares, "I believe we were not made with a spirit of fear. We have to break the barriers that fear confines us. In our daily lives if we are faced with two options, we need to get to the bottom of why we would NOT choose one of them. If the baseline for not choosing one of the options is fear, that is the one we should choose. I think that fear comes to us from an outside source, a darkness that tries to cover up the blessing. If we can push past that initial discomfort and choose to take a leap of faith, we can then experience the blessing."

So with that in mind, lets Get Radical and take these three ingredients (Radical Yes, Radical Opportunity in Adversity, and Radical Decision Making) and start the process of mixing them up. It is now time to take these potent components and add balance to them through creating a radical prescription that can be implemented and utilized in your own life.

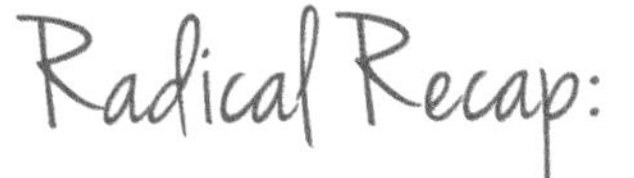

When you find yourself faced with a Radical Decision, always remember that:

1. Decisions often define who we are and outline the parameters through which we live our lives.
2. Good, bad, or indifferent, be a decision-maker.
3. Decision makers are truly difference makers.
4. The most successful people make the most decisions and the most mistakes.
5. Indecision is a dangerous mirage.
6. Own your decisions in the moment and acquire a talk track of empowerment.
7. Make radical decisions to move in the direction of your dreams.
8. Find yourself feeling indecisive? Focus on those times when you made a decision that changed your life. Then imagine if you didn't make that decision. Where would you be today?

Chapter 7:
RADICAL PASSION AND PURPOSE

Martyrs have given their lives for it.

True believers have sacrificed all they had to fulfill it.

Entrepreneurs risked the roof over their heads to accomplish it.

History celebrates those few that filled their lives with it.

Even thought-provokers reach the peak of greatness because of it.

Passion.

Purpose.

Small, two-syllable words with larger-than-life meaning. With passion and purpose, you can move mountains. Without it, you can barely even move.

Ralph Waldo Emerson told us that purpose should "make some difference that you have lived and lived well."

Robert F. Kennedy reminds us that the purpose of life "is to contribute in some way to making things better."

Robert Byrne said, "The purpose of life is a life of purpose."

But maybe the Dalai Lama serves our purpose best when he says, "Our prime purpose in this life is to help others." For us, this resounds the most.

The opportunities are vast and endless when your passion drives your purpose and your purpose drives your passion. The two play with one another in a harmonious and synchronistic way, culminating in what can only be described as something greater than the sum of its parts. The synergy is electric, the results genuine and authentic. No prescription is complete without a strong dose of passion and purpose.

RADICAL *thought*

Maintaining goals driven by passion and purpose resulting in specific and clear intention can often be the difference maker in your life and ultimately in the lives of others.

Liz: Passion is that indescribable thing that bubbles up inside of you that gives you unbounded energy to do whatever it takes, to meet whatever challenge, knowing there's a level of excitement because you're up to something that matters. Typically, it's bigger than you.

It leads you to a state of personal fulfillment and self-expression that makes you feel alive and connects you with others at a very core level. With passion, fatigue typically doesn't come into play because the energy that drives passion also provides a kind of everlasting, Energizer bunny-like battery that gets inserted into you and takes you wherever you need to go. No matter how late it is, how tired you are, how many countries you've traveled, you hook back into that ultimate source and it allows you to follow through and be passionate with purpose.

You feel the rush. It's something that you know and with which you are familiar. It resonates within your core. When we swing into that lane of being on our passion path, something really moves us from the inside and pushes us to share and give to others. That's when we wake up with energy and feel alive. It is like nothing will get in our way when we are in that lane. It's a real feeling. You don't have to talk about it and you don't have to convince anybody. You are it. You are in that moment of feeling fully alive and embraced and engaged in what it is that you are doing, and are excited by the impact you are leaving on a friend, family member, and possibly the world.

The truth is that purpose and passion are like a wildly burning fire within. One that cannot be tamed and is so hot that it keeps you heated and fueled throughout your journey. Simply put, the prescription for a radical life starts with that fire: being driven by purpose and passion.

Liz: When I was trying to find my passion path, it felt like a blur. I asked myself, what were some of the most impactful moments of my life?

Moments when I was unconsciously yet consciously at one and unaware of time while feeling really alive. Times when I could feel the energy pulse through me. Times when I simply felt beautiful. The moments that revealed themselves, although diverse, took on a theme of giving, sharing, and expressing myself authentically with others and making a difference. Moments of love, of design, of non-profit mission work in third-world countries, and a moment when I was asked to speak at the 3% Club by my friend and mentor Bob Proctor about my success.

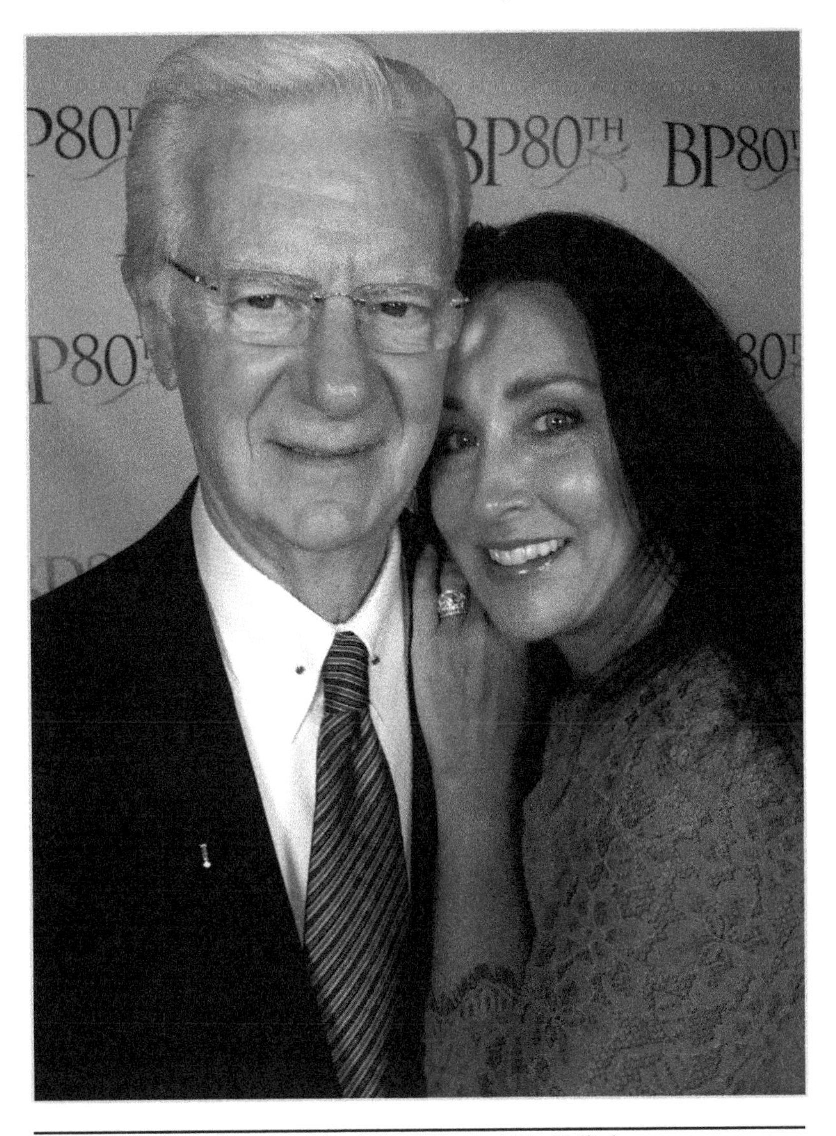

World Renowned Speaker Bob Proctor and Liz Edlich

The speaking engagement arrived on a truly challenging and traumatic day. A day in which I had to stand for what I believed in: I chose to fire my friend and the president of my company, tell the staff, shareholders, and investors that I had done it, and question if I was a living example of success at all.

Adversity and decision making had collided in the most resounding way, but my passion, purpose and commitment to give this presentation led me to the magical moment where I said YES and made the decision to speak in spite of the tears rolling down my cheeks as I made my way to the stage.

I looked out to see an ocean of faces that had just witnessed an impactful seminar and were wound up by one of the world's greatest speakers, Bob Proctor. His thunderous voice and unbridled energy and enthusiasm could be felt in the core of your body when he spoke. So there I was on stage, I had my star-studded two-minute video to open, I had my PowerPoint, I was dressed impeccably, and yet all I could think was, *who am I to talk about success today? I feel like a failure, bumped and bruised and unsure of tomorrow and the decisions I just made.*

I made my way onto the stage toward the end of my video, I steeled my gaze, and as I looked out before me, I knew I had no choice. I choked back the tears and decided to tell them the naked truth and jump into a pool of authenticity, hoping that maybe the wake of my fall would touch them. And that is how it began. For the most part, I threw out the PowerPoint and just spoke from the heart. I shared that even though I had achieved all that was in the brochure and onscreen, today I did not feel successful or worthy of the stage on which I stood. It was the ultimate impostor syndrome upfront and center.

As my story unfolded, I shared some of the tools I had learned on my business journey, some success models they could apply to their world, the challenges I had faced and currently faced, and what I had done and would do again to overcome them. Then something extraordinary happened. I felt alive. I was in a stream of consciousness sharing anything and everything I could think of to help those before me. I knew no time. I only knew a sense of love and giving in that moment. And I sensed that I uplifted those around me. There was an exchange of beautiful energy. And when I was finished I saw that many in the audience had tears in their eyes. When they clapped and stood to speak to me, I realized that I had in fact touched them by simply being authentic and accessible, and that made me beautiful. Creating more moments like this became my goal.

In that moment I realized that I had a glimpse of my passion, my purpose, and I would welcome living more radical moments in that suspended place of shared authenticity and motivational speaking with the intention of making a difference.

RADICAL *thought*

Authenticity is a necessary ingredient for helping others to feel beautiful.

That one snapshot of a forty-five-minute period of time, on a very difficult day of my life filled with adversity, became a glimpse of a passion hotspot that I have used again and again to keep my life rudder pointed in the direction of my radical fulfillment. That moment is one of my ingredients in the radical cake that Rachel and I have been baking together that takes us around the world to make a difference and to help others feel beautiful.

PASSION HOTSPOTS

Finding your passion and purpose is the next step. It takes inward reflection, evaluation, and asking questions.

Questions like:

- *What do I love to do?*
- *What gives me endless energy?*
- *What am I good at?*
- *What have I never tried but I have always dreamed of doing?*
- *What keeps me awake at night with a smile on my face?*
- *What lights me up in the morning when my eyes open?*
- *When do I feel in the flow, losing focus of time?*

Passion and purpose are grounded in living a full and all-out sort of life. It means doing more of what you love and maybe even expanding that circle of what you cherish into greater territory that you haven't yet experienced. We all have passion hotspots in our own lives that are expressed in activities, friendships, conversations, emotions, decisions, and even moments. Embrace these indicators you identify and look to expand on them.

RADICAL *thought*

Create a vision board with images that express your heart's desire. It will ignite what is possible, and your subconscious and conscious mind will conspire to create it. It is not about what you are trying to get, it is about what you are trying to grow.

These passion hotspots point us in the direction of a passionate and purposeful life. So it's really about taking the time to inwardly reflect and identify what really lights us up. Think of that moment and then ride the momentum of that moment recreating itself in numerous situations.

Dino Buccola, who died of Lou Gehrig's disease, was a close friend, an investment banker, and someone who taught us an enormous amount about business during the sweet spot of his career. But it was his battle with this rare disease that taught us more about life than we could ever imagine. While we watched him fight for his life, we decided that every Wednesday night we would gather our friends with his friends and family, and have dinner together and surround him with love, friendship, and laughter. We started this process to help him, but in the end we were the ones who benefited the most.

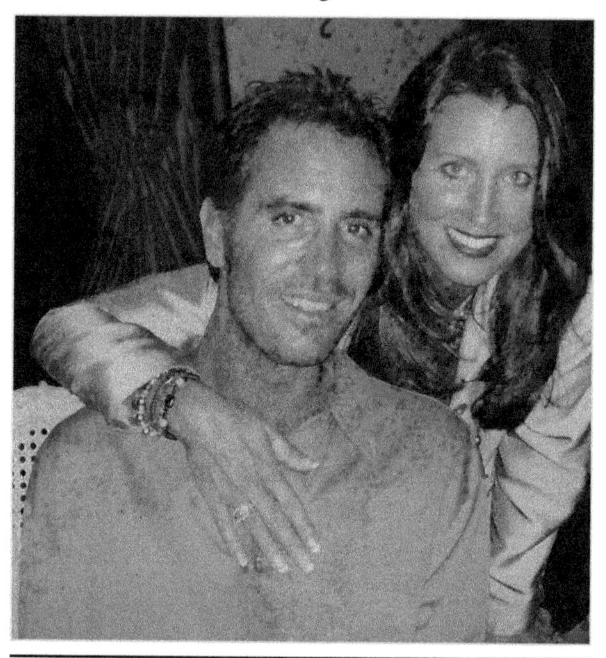

Dino & Liz at a Dino Knight gathering

Those of us who met over the years during our Wednesday night dinners, even around his bedside in the nursing home, built amazing friendships together, created connections, and exchanged passion and purpose. We took time out of our crazy busy lives to be there for another human being, and it was that experience that ended up transforming our lives. After these evenings, we felt rich as knights (which was a play on Dino nights; we even made hats that said "Dino Knights"). We would all sit around the table, tell stories, ask for advice, and disconnect from everything on the outside. In his last five years, Dino could only communicate through the slightest blink of his eyes, and he would painfully spell out each letter and each word on an alphabet card. But he was always aware, present, and locked in.

Rachel: After three or four years of assisted living, he fought to be alive in a nursing home while lying down watching TV 24/7. He communicated through blinking his eyes. Thinking about that reminds me how lucky I am every single day. I have so much gratitude for my health. You just can't take that for granted. When I think of challenges, when I think of obstacles, when I think of all those things, it's like, yeah, I deal with them, but sitting there with Dino put everything in perspective.

We remember watching him, immobile, sitting with us and noticing a sunset in the background. We asked him, "Dino, what would you say to all of us now, being where you are and looking back? What is your advice for living a radical life?"

RADICAL *thought*

"Every day I suggest that you get up and grab life between the ears and give it a big wet sloppy kiss." – Dino Buccola

We have never forgotten these words. Dino was an amazing teacher, and he gave us a perspective in his last days that our individual responsibility is to live a life of passion and purpose.

PEARLS AND PASSION

When asked about the key to living a life filled with passion, one of our best girlfriends, Yvette Mimeux, said, "Each moment is a pearl. As you string together these fabulous pearls, you realize that you suddenly have a beautiful necklace full of luster and brilliance that you can take with you everywhere."

In the end, it's the memories of moments well lived that count. The individual with the longest necklace wins in his or her life. So get off the bleachers and get out on the field and play. Play big, like your life depends on it, and share your beautiful necklace with those you love. And always remember to grab life by the ears and give it a big wet sloppy kiss.

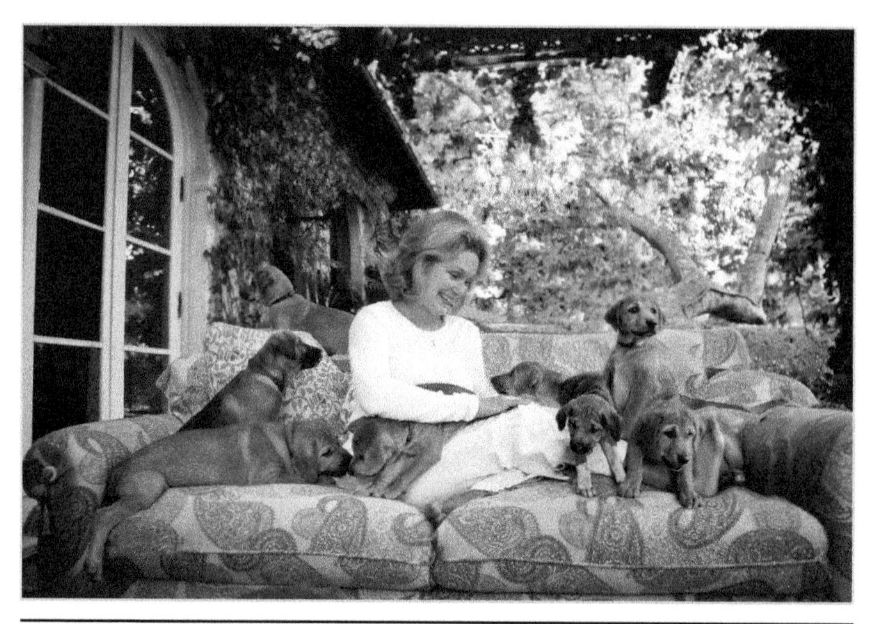

Yvette Mimeaux Ruby and her puppies

Darling Lizzy,

May your glass always be full. Half full is not interesting and half empty is not an option. All joy to you my beautiful friend, always with so much love.

Yvette

But don't just take our word for it, as there is plenty of scientific and quantitative support for the importance of living a purposeful and happy life. Just ask our friend Dan Buettner, who unequivocally found that a purposeful life actually helps you to live longer. Dan is an explorer, educator, public speaker, and most importantly, a friend. He is a *New York Times* bestselling author and National Geographic Fellow, and has delivered more than three thousand speeches to audiences worldwide. His TED Talk "How to Live to Be 100+" has been viewed over two million times. We spoke to him about the passion and purpose he noticed in people across the globe.

Dan told us, "For many people we encountered, they were fortunate enough to live in cultures where purpose was part of everyday vocabulary. It's a little different than the lives we have in America where we have to find our purpose. If you go to a place like Okinawa, Japan, they find meaning in their entire lives. They don't even have the word retirement. Instead, they just ask, 'What do I love to do?' And, almost more importantly: 'What is expected of me? What does the community expect of me that gets me up in the morning?' I just think that before you can do anything radical you need to get a clear sense of your values, what you like to do, what you're good at, and most importantly, how you can share them. Because keeping those gifts to yourself really doesn't do much good to anybody."

That is how we felt with Radical Skincare sitting on our counter and not out there working for you. It was doing no good sitting there. That is why we said, let's get on it and spread our passion and purpose to the world and see what good it can do.

So, if you are feeling caught in the hamster-wheel of life, the monotony of the norm, and the complacency of the same, join the crowd. This feeling is a worldwide epidemic. And there is a better life for the taking. There is more. It comes from knowing what your passion hotspots are and taking steps toward that which ignites you. That doesn't mean we have to make a big change to truly be radical. The prescription simply begins by welcoming, with open arms, the possibility to live a passionate and purposeful life.

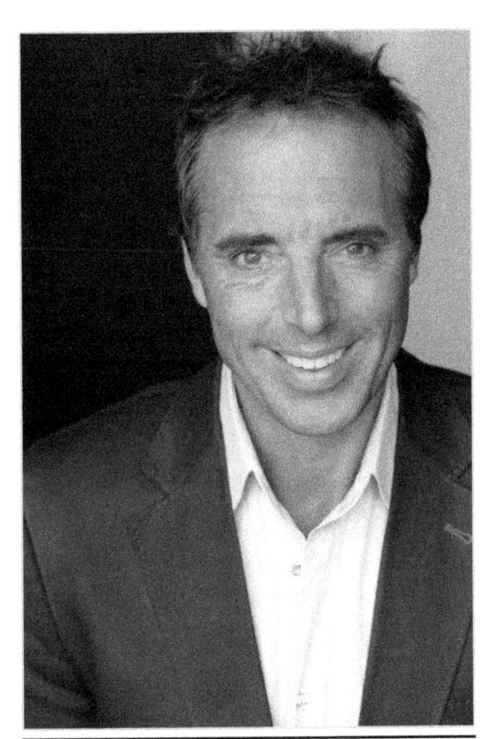

Author and Speaker Dan Buettner

As Dan Buettner told us, "Most Americans are doing work they don't like. I think they should switch jobs and do something they absolutely love to do, and forever. Unless you're severely disabled, you should be spending some of your day applying your gifts. That's what is going to keep you young, and it is what's going to give you the sense of fulfillment and contentment being a human being."

Radical means replacing "not today" with "today," trading "some other time" for "no other time," and swapping "maybe later" for "right now!"

The possibilities are endless. But they call for the desire to unleash and unlock your potential. That potential may have been buried by past experiences, relationships, and the bumps and bruises that life often inflicts. It is time to get up, dust off, and fight for a passionate and purposeful life. Radical people are driven by the P & P. And so are you. Now it is time to reclaim yours.

RADICAL *thought* | Use Passion and Purpose to radically reclaim what is yours!

Our friend Dyan Cannon is one of Hollywood's most celebrated and timeless leading ladies. Throughout her career, she has dedicated herself to her trade and has constantly been considered a versatile and talented artist. No matter what she does, she does it with 100 percent dedication and desire. And the manner in which she loves is no different.

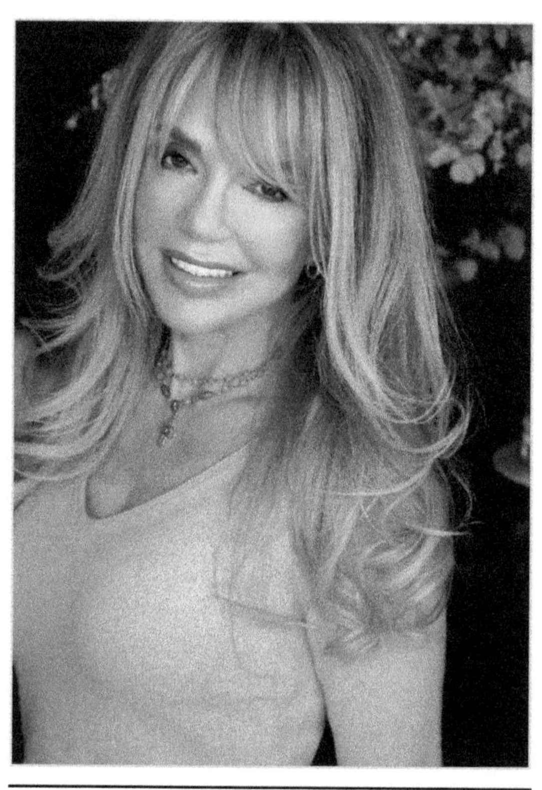

Actress Dyan Cannon

When we spoke, she reminded us of the relationship between passion and fear. "I think the thing that would limit our passion is fear. The fear that we won't succeed, that the other person won't love us back, that we won't make it. That we're too fat, too thin, too young, or too old. When we take those limits off and choose to live a life with love instead of fear, then passion can bloom. You can't make passion. If you're not passionate, you can't make it. But you can learn how to live it by taking off the limits in your life. The only way you can remove the limits is by getting the limiting self out of the way, and the only way to get yourself out of the way is to go to a higher power."

So when people ask us, "Where do we start?" the answer is an easy one. The prescription for living a radical life is substantially based on maintaining an inspired and purpose-driven attitude. We want to help you get back to what you love. What you forgot. What you remember but let slip away. Or simply what you know you are capable of.

Why?

Because *you* said so.

You need no permission to be radical, to embrace your full potential and possibility. You need only to say the *Radical Yes.* That energy alone sets everything that you desire in motion.

RADICAL TRANSFORMATION

Our friend of twenty years, Cynthia Kersey, is a shining example of the power of radical transformation. In fact, she is a pioneer in the transformational industry. Her two bestselling books, *Unstoppable* and *Unstoppable Women,* contain a myriad of inspiring stories and strategies from people all over the globe who overcame obstacles to reach success. Cynthia is now the chief humanitarian officer of the Unstoppable Foundation, "whose mission is to ensure that every child on the planet receives access to the life-long gift of education."[4] Cynthia has always been a huge inspiration to us, and for years she urged us to write *Get Radical.* We watched her radically transform her own life, and in the process change the lives of countless others.

"There are many components to my story that would be considered radical or unstoppable," Cynthia told us. "Before I wrote the book, I worked for Sprint, which as you know is a large corporation. I started from the bottom as an entry-level telemarketer and went on to become a national account manager making six figures. However, I wasn't passionate about my life. I had always loved stories about unstoppable people. Even though I'd never written anything more than a college term paper, in 1996 I downsized my life and cashed in my entire life savings to write my first book, *Unstoppable.* The book came out and now I'm living a more purposeful life, which is to inspire people to also live an unstoppable life, like I had been inspired by these stories.

"Two months after the book came out, my twenty-year marriage ended. I called my mentor, Millard Fuller, and he said, 'When you have a great pain in your life, you need a greater purpose.' He had just gotten back from Nepal, and he said, 'Why don't you build a house for a family in need?' As I thought about his advice, I questioned how many houses I would need to build to offset the pain in my life."

Cynthia continued, "Even though I was living a purposeful life – I had left a corporate job to write the book and speak with people – it wasn't bigger than my pain. That year, when I was out there speaking and grieving and healing, I started the Unstoppable Nepal Project or Nepal Build. I raised $200,000 and a year later took eighteen people to Nepal, and we worked on the first three of the one hundred homes that were subsequently built. It wasn't until we got to one hundred houses that it started to offset my pain.

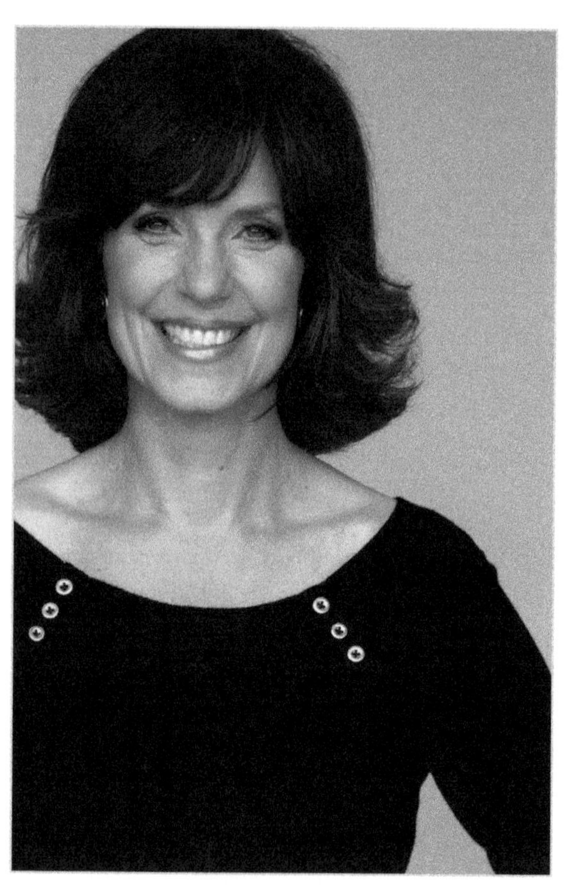

Unstoppable Foundation Founder and Author Cynthia Kersey

"That trip was a very pivotal experience for me, because while I initially thought I was doing something big for the Nepalese people, I hadn't anticipated what it would do for me personally. I connected with them and felt the power of giving in a way I had never before experienced. What was interesting was that that year I made more money than I had earning a six-figure income, yet that wasn't my intention. Everything just worked out, and I feel that the story is a great representation of the power of giving.

"My second book, *Unstoppable Women,* came out in 2005. I was invited to go to this rural African women's conference. The only thing I knew about this conference was that women were coming to share their stories. That's it. I knew one person who was going, and I couldn't shake the feeling that I should absolutely go.

"Last minute I rearranged my schedule, flew over there, and met four hundred women, many of whom had walked for days, and miles and miles and miles, sometimes with babies on their backs, to meet with us and share their stories – not from a place of victimhood, but truly from a place of empowerment. They were saying, 'We need to get our kids clean water. How do we treat our children that are dying from malaria?' The number one thing they said was, 'How do we get our kids an education?' because without it nothing will change. And so I fell in love with them. I promised them I would do something. I had no idea what it would be, and quite frankly their situation seemed overwhelming to me. I didn't even know how they could possibly be so positive in light of their circumstances.

I came home, started doing some research, and really understood that education is the key. It's the fundamental element to helping people lift themselves out of poverty. "For me, I think the best way to be radical or unstoppable is to find a purpose that's bigger than you. I, personally, have never been motivated by money. I'm motivated by what that money can do. When I look at it that way, I am always inspired. As I look at my life, inspiration is the key; so I would ask, for all people wanting to be radical, what inspires you? What is that calling within you that lights you up and doesn't feel like a chore or an obligation? When I talk about giving, I'm really talking from a place of inspiration, from a place of sheer joy. When you find that, it will not only transform other people's lives, but it will completely and radically transform your life as well."

Cynthia was able to connect with a larger purpose – one that positioned her to transform the lives of countless others. Her journey has just begun as she continues to make a difference by pursuing her passion and purpose through sharing the opportunity of giving with others via her Unstoppable Foundation.

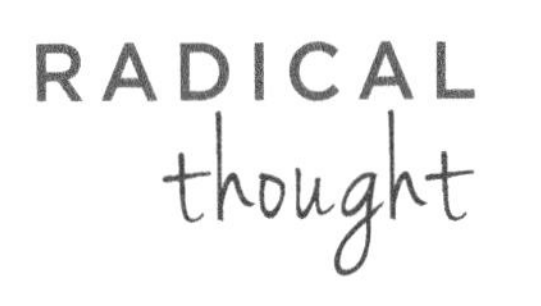

Take the time each and every day of your life to identify your passion and purpose and then go get it. The result will be something beautiful, exciting, and stunning.

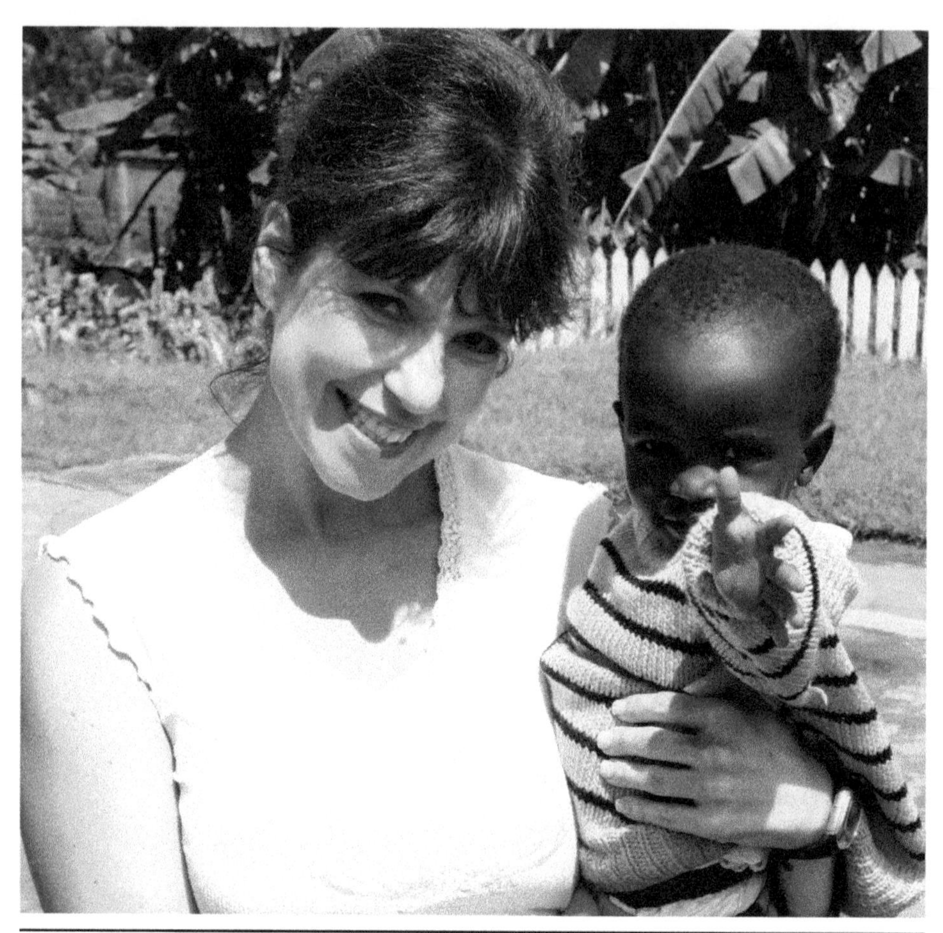

Cynthia Kersey, with one of her Unstoppable Foundation kids, Unstoppablefoundation.org

Nelson Mandela said, "There is no passion to be found playing small – in settling for a life that is less than the one you are capable of living." Radical is a go-big or go-home kind of life. That doesn't mean every swing has to be for the fences, but it does mean that every moment, every day, every decision, and every opportunity is respected, cherished, and moved by passion and purpose.

Radical Recap:

When you find yourself running low on passion and purpose, always remember that:

1. Maintaining goals driven by passion and purpose can often be the difference maker in your life and ultimately in the lives of others.

2. The opportunities are vast and endless when your passion drives your purpose and your purpose drives your passion.

3. Passion means doing more of what you love and maybe even expanding that circle of what you cherish into greater territory that you haven't yet experienced.

4. Passion and purpose can break down barriers that stand taller than you, feel stronger than you, and look impenetrable to you.

5. Radical means replacing "not today" with "today," trading "some other time" for "no other time," and swapping "maybe later" for "right now!"

6. When you have a great pain in your life, you need a greater purpose driven by passion.

7. Always remember to grab life by the ears and give it a big wet sloppy kiss.

8. Passion and purpose lead you to your destiny.

9. Passion and purpose create a life worth living.

Chapter 8:
RADICAL VISUALIZATION

Important to creating a prescription for living a radical life is your desire to build a radical vision. To do so, you have to imagine the outcome that you desire. Radical requires you to think just a little outside of the box. It inspires you to feel just a little uncomfortable and take risks that you may not ordinarily take. A radical life is one that is logical and careful, but also one that is willing to suspend disbelief, get dirty by uncovering every stone, and one that is ready to jump into the rabbit hole into the unknown.

Radical pushes you to be different because different can be the difference.

See it and believe it, so you can visualize and own it. At times it can be as simple as that. George Bernard Shaw said, "Imagination is the beginning of creation."

For us, it started with imagination. Imagination often acted as the lubricant for us to create a skincare line, to live a radical life, and then to take those lessons and experiences we learned along the way and offer them to you. Imagination is about having no boundaries.

Think about your own childhood, or if you are now a parent, how your children interact with the world around them. Children are a riveting and mesmerizing example of wonder. They have an endless ability to lose themselves in the fantasy they create. They are not worried about those around them or the reactions they may receive. Rather, they are lost in the endless world of opportunity.

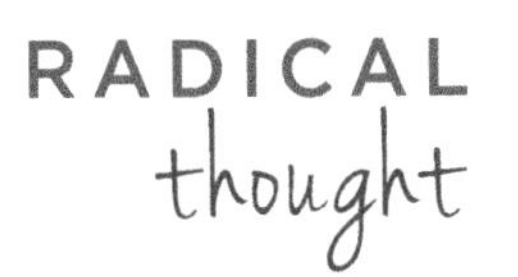

Radical people turn down the volume of the nay-sayers and turn up the volume of the dreamers.

Imagine your goals and then set aside logic to move toward your purpose.

For us, imagination lives in the "beyond possible" area of life. To live a radical life and truly elevate your happiness, you really have no choice but to slam on the brakes, take a hard right turn, and set up shop at the corner of imagination lane.

Radical people are focused. They develop that higher side of their personality. They develop their imagination. Imagination gives them the ability to bring the future into the present and live with it in their mind until it manifests in form. That's where all creation leads us.

And much like our skincare line, science is an important factor to learn from to create the success you want, and have a statistically shorter road to getting there. To that point, most scientists agree that nothing was ever accomplished without imagination. We may just be imagining that statistic, but that statement isn't all that far from the truth.

RADICAL *thought*

Albert Einstein advises that "to stimulate creativity, one must develop the childlike inclination for play." [5]

More and more, imagination is not only being studied but also supported in the scientific community as a leading indicator of success. In fact, well-respected and trained scientists are dedicating their lives to studying the mind and its interaction with the outside world to better understand how imagination creates action and results.

Jim Davies, PhD, is a cognitive scientist, associate professor, and the director of the Science Imagination Laboratory at Carleton University. He says, "Imagination keeps us going. Sometimes, as adults, we lose the ability to imagine because we're in the daily grind of being grownups. And then you walk into your home and are grabbed by your child and whisked away into a magical fairytale land where anything is possible. Those moments should serve as reminders that you have the ability to incorporate that childlike energy into your daily life and unleash the creativity, and live life without boundaries."

RADICAL *fact*

According to a study by Dr. Stephanie Carlson at the University of Minnesota, children spend nearly two-thirds of their time in imaginative play. [6]

As young children, it is socially acceptable to be daydreamers, to be creative, to be energetic and passionate. In fact, most of our educators would push us to color outside the lines.

But as we mature, after the ripe old age of five, we are taught that when coloring:

- Leaves are green.
- The sun is yellow.
- The sky is blue.
- And make sure you do your best to color within the lines.

That simple teaching and behavior becomes a metaphor for our entire lives. It hampers our ability to create our own reality. The truth is that it is the unbridled moments to color outside the lines that actually breathe life into passion and progress.

Rachel: I have noticed that when I was a kid, and now with my children, there is pressure in society to color in the lines, follow directions, and take the cookie cutter approach to get from point A to point B. This starts when most of us are in school, and we are scrutinized. If we miss a milestone, it brings on the feelings of inadequacy. For the first five years of life, we are encouraged to live in imagination land, be creative and fully self-expressed. We are applauded for our first word, step, dance, song; we live fully and learn in every moment and disappear into a world of imagination that has no limits.

You were not thinking of next week or next year, but rather were being truly present in the moment. This is soon suppressed when you enter school with structure and are pushed to fit in and follow expected behavior. You are taught to drive for academics and are expected to conform to what society and parents say are the best ways to be successful in life. The pressure starts building and we lose that feeling of freedom to dream big. As an adult, fear of failure, of not being enough, of not deserving success, an aversion to risk, worry, a sense of responsibility, and a lack of confidence begin to knock on the door of life, and you think that where you are supposed to be. You don't push the envelope, and you get uncomfortable with dreaming big.

You have to change that conversation and tap back into visualization, knowing that you deserve to have a life you love. Commit to creating the magic and self-expression in your life every day. Ignite your own childlike imagination and creativity to construct a life you love. Visualization and imagination have no boundaries!

Therefore, we firmly believe life should be lived at the intersection of fun and possibility. A radical life is a boundless one. It is as infinite as the ocean, as vast as space, and as bright as the most visible star in the sky. Imagine the life you want. Visualize the goals for which you reach.

RADICAL *thought*

Being in action creates results. Paint a picture in your mind of what happiness looks and feels like to you. Give yourself the freedom to start with a new palette, and even if it's make-believe, create what it would look like. Start getting emotionally involved, because if you're going to do something, you might as well be fully invested.

THE ART OF VISUALIZATION

Visualization is one of the most powerful tools that we will give you in this book. It can look and feel like child's play, but frankly there is nothing more powerful. If you are hell-bent and determined to create a radical and magical world that excites you, visualization is one of the keys that we implore you to adopt. The time is *now.*

Okay, here we go.

Take a few moments to locate some magazines or images off of the Internet that light you up. Find a white board and scissors and glue sticks. Build a collage that represents your dreams. Look to travel magazines, money magazines, Women's or Men's Health, Oprah magazine, Bride, family magazines and many more. Cut out pictures and images or words that represent what you like. See yourself there and visualize how it feels, smells, and looks. The list is your list and yours alone. Have fun and Get Radical.

Why do this exercise?

Why create a collage of pictures that reflects your dream to create your desired reality? Because your subconscious mind holds tight to the paradigms of yesterday, and your reality of tomorrow suffers because of it.

The subconscious mind works in images. For example, if I say dog, you don't see D-O-G as in the letters. You think of the image of a dog, whatever that may be. If I say your living room, you picture your living room and probably can see most of the things that are in it and how they are situated. You do not see L-I-V-I-N-G R-O-O-M as letters spelled out. Therefore, when you adopt and get emotionally involved with an image, you are on your way to creating it because your subconscious mind already believes that you have it. You begin to energetically vibrate in this frequency, and sure enough you start to attract all that is needed for you to make that vision possible. We have so many examples and evidence of this that are indisputable. Visualization is one of the most important steps to creating a life you love and bringing it to fruition.

So for a moment suspend reality, and realize that anything is possible.

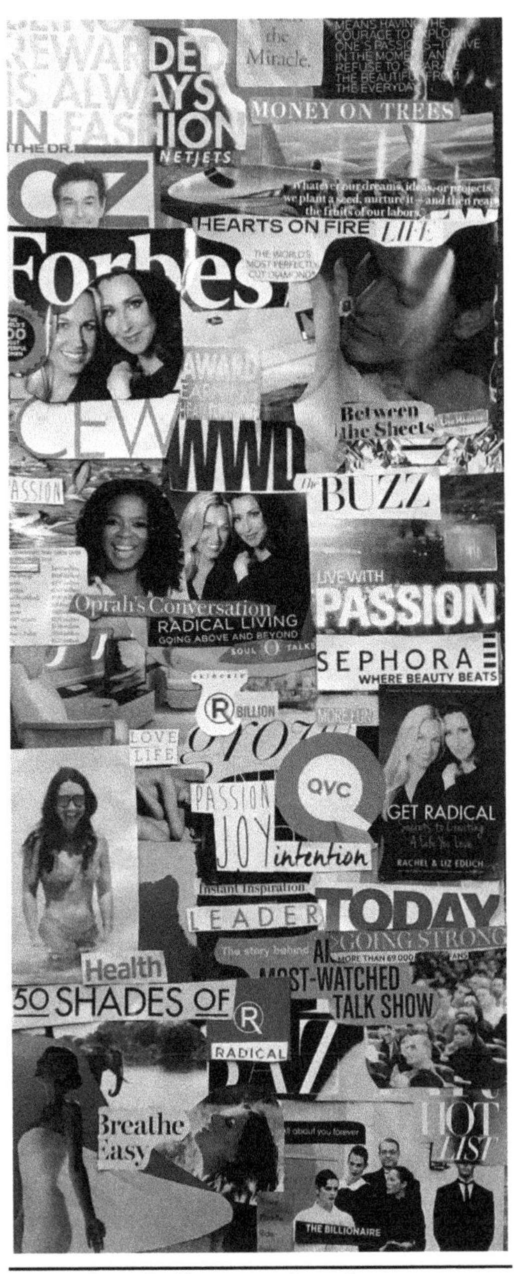

Liz and Rachel's Vision Board

Lift the heavy dark ceilings of hopelessness and disbelief and give yourself permission to suspend your perceived reality and visualize your hearts' desires.

Miracles have occurred in our life through visualization – creating a vision of what is possible because you hold an image in your mind. It must be clear and defined and represent your dreams and you must be emotionally involved.

Liz: I am proof that this dream board visualization process really works. Rachel and I were filming Bob Proctor for *The Power to Have it All* TV series that we created together. In the process of filming we had to interview people that had followed his principles and practiced them. Person after person showed us their goal cards and their vision board and told us their stories. After months of interviews and filming, Rachel and I came to the conclusion that this goal setting vision board process was as close to having the keys to getting what you want as anything else out there. So we did it ourselves.

On my vision board I had a boat, and an exotic island home with tree trunks as the corners with white sheers blowing in the windows. I had a picture of our fly-fishing lodge that I was hoping we would sell and so I printed out a picture of the lodge and put a sold sign on it with a dollar amount. I cut out a picture of a hot guy lifting weights from Men's Health and put a picture of my husband's face over his face. I put a dollar amount on the board that I wanted in the bank. I cut out logos of QVC, television shows, Forbes, a picture of me and Rachel speaking in front of thousands of people inspiring them with words like inspiration, passion, buzz, grow, health, and love. The below story is just one example of my visualization coming to fruition.

What if I told you that stopping a Vespa in front of a random house for no other reason than a gut instinct would dramatically change my life? This impulsive moment has led me to visiting the island of Tahiti numerous times in the last ten years, creating a new world of friendships and more joy than I ever imagined, all because of visualization, intuition and doing something crazy without a seemingly logical reason. Intuition and visualization are keys that unlock the door to a life of living your dreams.

I believe visualization and intuition are two of the most important factors in having everything that you desire. The little clues that take you off your mapped-out route lead you to your riches. Riches can be more than just money. They can be your relationships and friendships, or a job that you are passionate about. The list is endless.

What I marvel about is how important it is to listen to that little voice inside you, so you can be open to it and allow it to take you down those magical roads. There are books written about it, and there are numerous CEOs and athletes who attribute their success to following their intuition and visualizing.

For me, the best example is a trip I took with my husband to Tahiti over ten years ago. I had been once before, and I was drawn to French Polynesia. The people, the music, the mountains, the sea, and the French food didn't hurt this attraction either.

We went to a little island called Tahaa. It is an island less traveled to than Bora Bora or Moorea. There are no airports, no fancy hotels, just large Tahitian guesthouses for families, one small bed and breakfast, and a tiny island with a very nice Relais & Chateaux where we were staying.

As luck would have it, it decided to rain. When it rains in Tahiti, it can go on for days! After the third day of rain, I was researching flights to travel to places with the promise of sun. Finally the rain stopped. My husband and I decided to take the Vespa and explore the main island of Tahaa in search of the infamous pearl farms and a pearl, which was to be my reward for my interminable patience waiting out the rain.

With the sun kissing the land and trees, everything had a magical quality to it. On our journey to the end of the island and the pearl farm, about midway through I saw a house on the water that was open air, using tree trunks for the corners, with a very tropical yet different design from the other houses we passed. I told my husband to stop the Vespa because I wanted to see who owned it and who the designer was. At the time I had an interior design company in Malibu and was keenly interested in what inspired people to build what they build.

Dale responded, "Are you crazy? You cannot just stop at a complete stranger's house." But something inside me said it would be okay. I love adventure. What was the worst thing that could happen? After all, I felt compelled to stop. Dale carried on and drove past, ignoring my plea. He wrote it off as one of my impulsive moments, one of those moments that are hard to explain because from the outside they make little sense.

We continued down the road, arriving at the pearl farm, and asked to speak to the owner. Apparently, he had been taken to the hospital with a heart problem and thus the pearl farm was closed. So I was forced back on my Vespa, having completed the length of the island without a reward. On the way back, I begged Dale to stop while I pounded on his back like a child throwing a tantrum. He reluctantly pulled over to indulge my moment. Around the corner there was a young boy yelling, "You wanna see some pearls?" in his adorable French accent.

"Yes," I blurted out and said, "told you so" to Dale, so he could hear my triumph. Tama, the boy's father, offered us a Heineken, which I took even though I don't drink beer. The Radical Yes in action! I was up for the full adventure. We chatted and looked at pearls, finding a string of gorgeous aqua green pearls that I was considering taking. He told us to take the strand back to our hotel to "see how I like it." I asked him if he wanted my credit card information. He refused my card, saying, "I trust you." I thought to myself, *who does that? What planet is he on?*

So we took the strand with promises to return after living with it for a day. We went back to our hotel and spent the night discussing how refreshing this trusting way of living was. The next day we returned to Tama's home and at his insistence went snorkeling and ate at a local restaurant.

The following day we returned for more island fun and watched him free dive and spear fresh fish, which he then cooked on a wheelbarrow with coral and wood, using a screen as a grate to keep the fish from falling through. It went on like this for the next four days. We never returned to our hotel to eat again. We dove right into their family, their culture, and the generous spirit that they shared, and fell in love with them and the magic of French Polynesia.

As we were getting ready to leave the island and return to LA, we said our goodbyes at their house and of course bought our strand of pearls. I looked up at the mountain behind their house on the water and told them how beautiful it was. I had been watching the stars litter the sky night after night with that majestic hill as a backdrop. Tama and his wife, Virginie, informed us that they owned the land and had a dream to build a guesthouse and residence one day. Unfortunately, they said they thought they would never build it because it was too expensive. We looked at Tama and Virginie and said, "We'll build it." They stared back in disbelief with tears in their eyes.

It was their dream, but it was also mine. I longed to live in a culture as untouched as this and experience this type of island life. Within two weeks we had wired the money and the building began. Within four months our bungalow was built and we were staying there. Never a contract or scrap of paper changed hands. They gave us the land, we gave them the building and embarked on an adventure we named Tiare Breeze. Tiare is the name of the fragrant gardenia-like flower of Tahiti.

They rent the bungalow out to help support their family, and we bring friends and family to stay and vacation. Since that original meeting, we built an overwater pontoon and bought a boat to explore surf spots to snorkel and swim with the whales, which I did for almost half an hour with a mother and her calf less than fifty feet away! We hike, bike, eat, and have a group of local friends that we just love and adore.

The story and the magic only get better. A year later, I was moving my office and I took my vision board off my wall to pack away. As I looked over this glorified collage of things I wanted in my life, I was shocked to see before me a picture that I had cut out of a magazine. It was of an island bungalow with tree trunks supporting the corners and branches holding up the thatched roof. It looked just like what we had built in Tahiti. There was also a picture of a motorboat racing through the water. I was stunned. I realized that I had attracted and built my dream. I remembered making this collage and thinking that we couldn't afford another house, and I even wondered what I needed with a boat. But after seeing how many others had done these vision boards and experienced magical results, I did it and hung it in my office. To top it off our fly-fishing Lodge sold within 10 % of the price that I had written down; Rachel and I had been traveling around the world on stage and speaking to hundreds of people about passion and purpose; we did an interview for Forbes; and to top it off my husband began lifting weights.

All of this took place because of goal setting, my vision board, my intuition, and setting my intention on a dream. At the time I did not know "how" it would happen, I just knew it would. Think of the odds – because we are not French, we could not have legally purchased the land or afforded it in French Polynesia, but instead it was given to us. We got a boat that we have fondly named *Radical Gal.* All of these circumstances collided to deliver a dream. One that has given me wonderful memories and created so many friendships that span the years. A whole new life was available, a radical adventure, new friends and family because of a simple exercise in faith, intuition, and holding a vision.

Say the *Radical Yes* to following your intuition and creating the backdrop for your dreams.

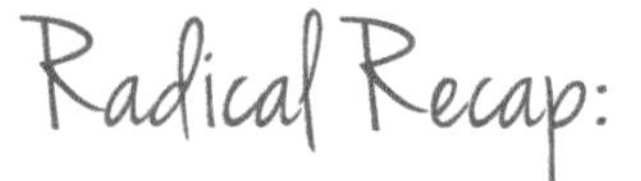

When visualizing a radical outcome, always remember that:

1. A radical life is one that is logical and careful, but also one that is willing to suspend belief. Be willing to jump into the rabbit hole and into the unknown.

2. Ignite your childlike creativity and visualize what you want.

3. Get emotionally involved with your vision. Become fully invested in your vision.

4. Imagine the life you want. Visualize the goals for which you reach. Then make them a reality.

5. Create the vision board of your dreams. Wake up to it and go to bed after looking at it. Play the movie in your mind when you wake up and go to sleep. It will then remain etched in your mind for you to attract.

6. Take a moment in the morning and before you sleep to see the vision of what you desire. Make it real in your mind and get emotionally involved in it.

7. You do not need to know HOW it will occur, just know that it will and that by holding your vision in your subconscious mind, you will attract all that is necessary to create it.

8. The power of visualization is strong. It is infinite, deep, and profoundly powerful. Don't overlook such an easy but potent opportunity.

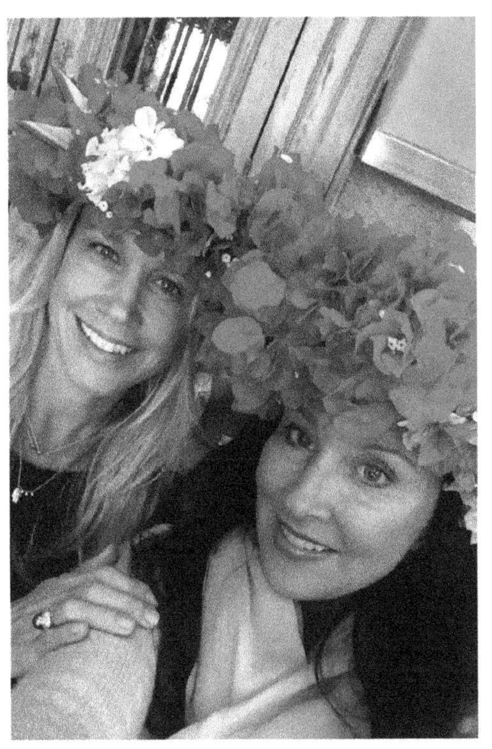

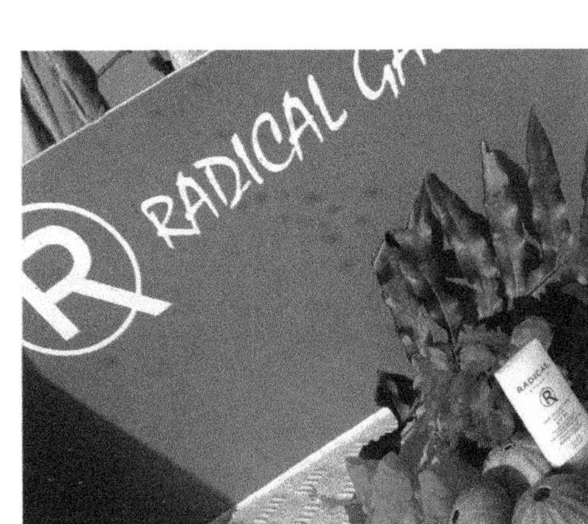
RADICAL

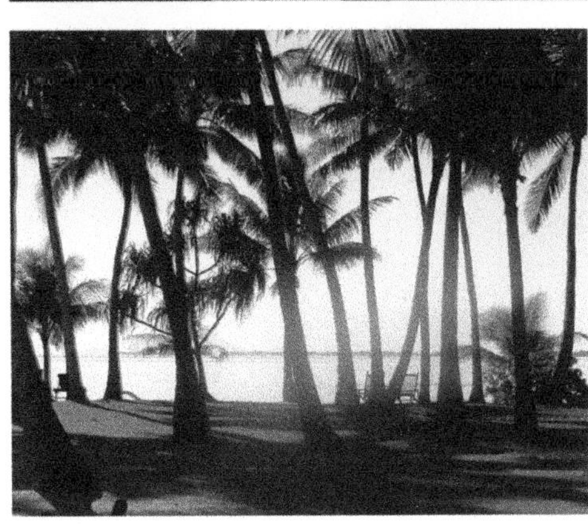

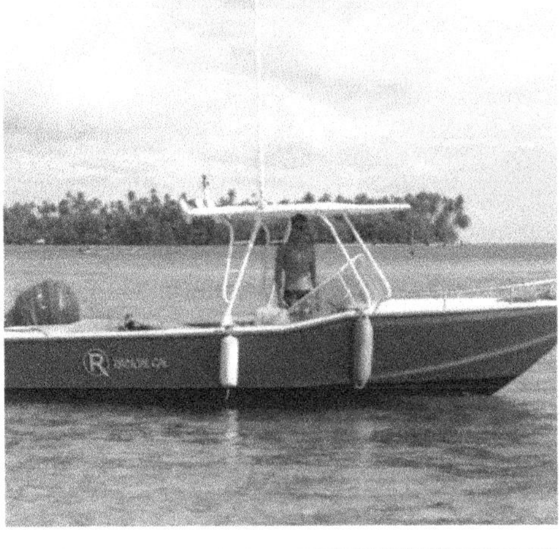

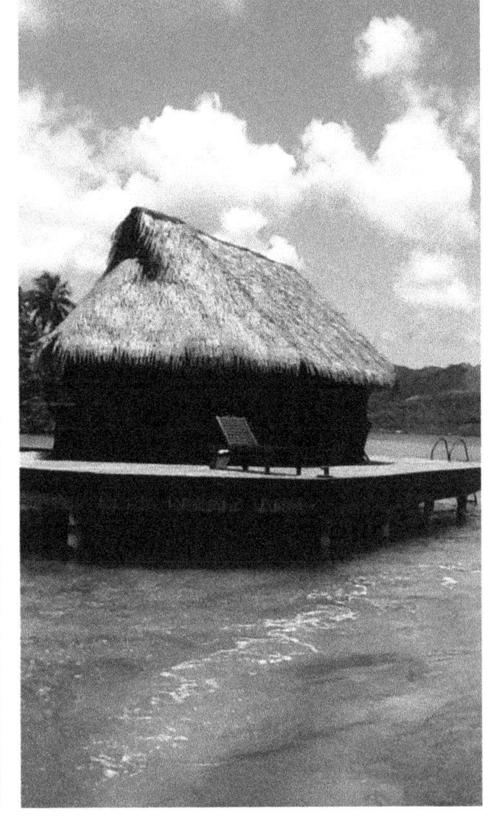

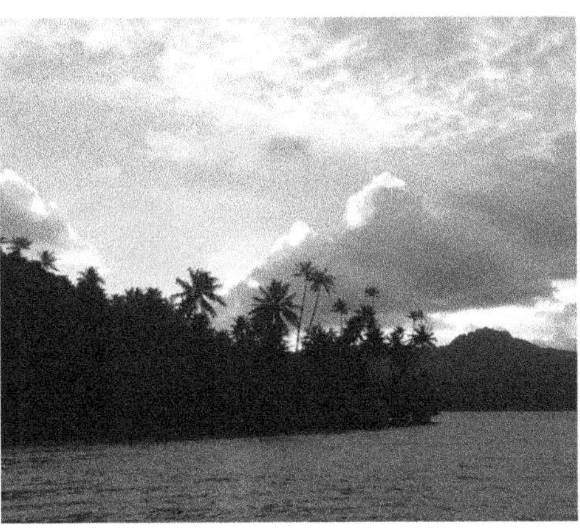

Chapter 9:
RADICAL OPPORTUNITY

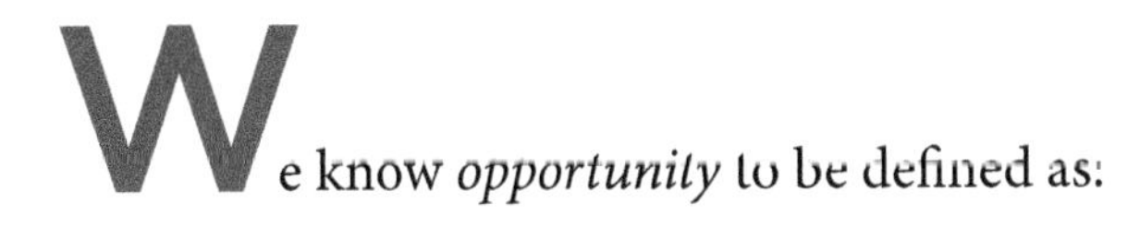

We know *opportunity* to be defined as:

A favorable juncture of circumstances;

A good chance for advancement or progress.

With our skincare line, it started as personal opportunity to fix our skin, but the knocks grew louder that there was more. As we shared our special formulas for skincare, we saw that there was an opportunity to formulate a prescription for life. It was there that our energy and instinct pushed us forward.

It wasn't our intention, but it clearly became our calling.

Think about it.

How many times have you experienced a full-steam-ahead journey that culminated in an entirely different outcome than you originally anticipated?

Opportunities are often redefined and transformed. They start in one form and then change into an entirely different one. Opportunity is not always respectful of your time, your energy, or your goals. It pretty much comes whenever it wants. But how you respond to it is a choice all your own. We can all agree that opportunity is an exciting endeavor. It makes your insides flutter, your heart beat just a little faster, and it often releases endorphins and elevates your mood.

But then all of a sudden your old paradigm and negative talk track kicks in and logic whispers in your ear.

It says things like:

- *Are you sure this is worth the risk?*
- *What if you fail?*
- *You don't have the education or experience to do that.*
- *What makes you think that you can do this in such a competitive world?*
- *What will people think if it doesn't work?*

These are the questions that often stifle opportunity, hold you captive, and cage you in while opportunity moves on to the next person.

But what if we viewed opportunity in a different light?

What if we assessed it through another lens?

The truth is that the way we view and assess opportunity is often the difference between seizing it and allowing it to pass us by. And make no mistake: not all opportunity is good opportunity. But the key is assessing the prospect before it passes you by.

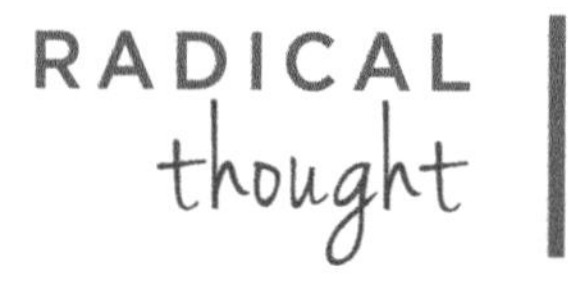

Everything has an element of risk. There are no guarantees in life. Try to push beyond the limits and put yourself in uncomfortable situations so that you know you are growing. Challenge the person you are today.

So what are the secrets to evaluating an opportunity before us?

1. ***Energy:*** *How your body feels toward the opportunity.*

   We humans are a whole bunch of vibrating energy. We vibrate high sometimes, we vibrate low at other times, but we are always vibrating. That vibration is often based on past experiences and journeys. Take the time to feel your energy and the energy of the opportunity before you decide to act or not act on it. Close your eyes and evaluate how your body feels when you think about it. Note the fear, but also recognize that the fear may be excitement in disguise, or just the fear of doing something different. Regardless, dig deep and trust your gut to guide you in the right direction.

2. **Instinct:** *How your gut reacts regarding the opportunity.*

   Some of your best decisions are probably based on instinct and something that you inherently feel. Like a hunch. It's the thing we all know exists but many times don't listen to. Instinct is the key to having that unexplainable edge that can open doors to great opportunities, even when you are initially unsure how or why.

3. **Intellect:** *How your mind analyzes the opportunity.*

   Decision making can be compared to a typical decision tree of pros versus cons. Look at what's written. Weigh the good and the bad. Do your best to be process oriented and fact specific because that kind of thinking doesn't have as many variables wrapped around it. This is where intellect meets opportunity. Educate yourself to expand your examples; notice patterns that you repeat and what works and what doesn't so as to not replicate unhealthy choices and support the wolves in sheep's clothing. The best way to do this is to take the time to review your thought process from past decisions to aid in a current situation. Jot down notes from your decision making process and do so with the intent that they may help you in the future.

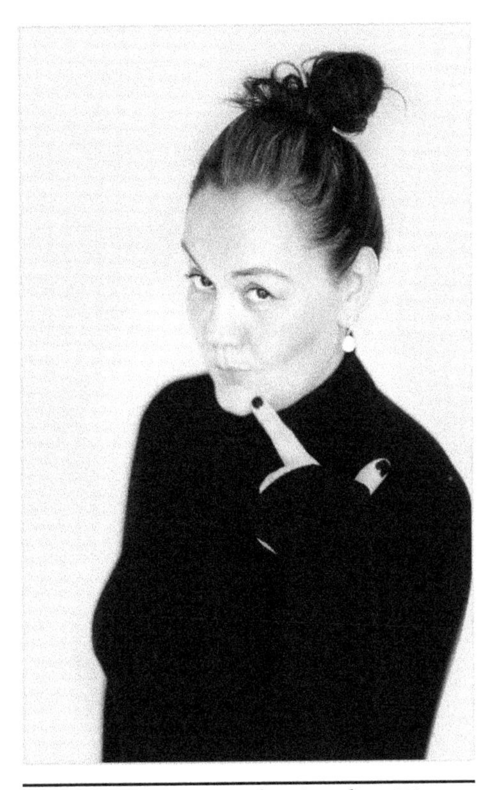

Beauty Industry Insider Caroline Hirons

Caroline Hirons is a third generation beauty industry insider. Consulting for numerous companies today she shares her passion for expressing your authentic self in life and in beauty with her blog. When Caroline is coaching or mentoring up-and-coming beauty bloggers, many times they will ask her: "What do you think I should do about the opportunity before me?" She asks them, " What does your gut tell you to do?" They often respond that their gut tells them yes but their agent tells them no. Caroline says, "Well you sleep with your gut, not your agent, so go for it. Speak your mind, stand for what you believe, and be your authentic self." Caroline follows her gut instinct in most areas of her life, from raising her children, to career, to love, and to friendships. She says your gut is spot on, so follow it and you wont be sorry.

At the end of the day, opportunities can be measured through the balancing of energy, instinct, and intellect. The culmination of the three will help you to analyze what stands before you. A radical life is one grounded in the notion of possibility. Each and every opportunity has a possibility within it to do something truly radical. As we developed our formula for success both inside and outside of the bottle, we tried our best to understand how we evaluated and then acted on the opportunities that knocked on our door.

RADICAL *thought*

Evaluate opportunities with a balance of energy, instinct, and intellect.

OUR RADICAL OPPORTUNITY

Life presents us with a multitude of opportunities in both our personal lives and in business. Our most glaring opportunity of late has been creating Radical Skincare. Sharing this exciting adventure together as sisters, we have had the unique opportunity to merge our passion on numerous levels with a business that brings us and others joy. But the opportunity came to us by surprise.

Seizing the opportunity to create a personal skincare solution for ourselves was an easy decision. Remember, we had a personal need that was not otherwise fulfilled on the market. So we set sail. And eventually we reached our destination. We healed our skin. That voyage was based on a personal need and motivation. But what came after was truly unexpected. We hadn't set sail to create a Radical Skincare line to sell. That was never even on our radar. But again, opportunity began to tap, then knock, then slam on our door. So we suspended reality and jumped into the rabbit hole. We answered the calling. And the results were electric. Radical Skincare led us on this radical journey and taught us how to live a radical life.

All opportunity should be welcomed. Meaning, when it knocks, crack the door open and see who is there.

The next step is to scrutinize the opportunity using your energy, instinct, and intellect to ensure it is the best fit for you. Radical people are those who love the potential for opportunity, but also carefully choose. That doesn't mean you can't live in the moment and seize the day, it just means you use the skills and characteristics that life experiences, successes, and failures have gifted you. Opportunity hides around each and every corner. Keep your eyes open and always be willing to actually turn the corners and peak into the crevices to see what is hiding in the dark. It takes a little effort, but in the end, you never know when that little expenditure of energy will make all the difference in your life.

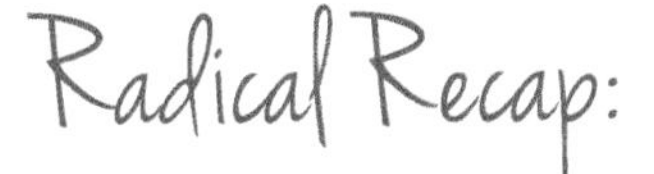

To invite radical opportunity into your own life, always remember that:

1. Opportunity is the culmination of energy, instinct and intellect. These are all gifts you've been given to help you maximize opportunity.

2. Opportunities are often redefined and transformed. They start in one form and then change into an entirely different one. Keep your eyes open.

3. Good, bad, or indifferent, opportunity is there for keeps. Remain open minded towards any prospect that comes your way. Everything happens for a reason and every opportunity should be assessed, evaluated, and considered.

4. Pay attention to how your body feels when an opportunity presents itself. Many times it will give you the feedback that you need to make a decision.

5. Your gut instinct is your friend and should be listened to.

Chapter 10:
RADICAL MENTORS

Living a radical life is never accomplished in a vacuum. Our prescription to create the radical life of your dreams is based on a willingness to teach and be taught; to learn and educate others; to listen but also talk; and to carefully choose the people with whom you surround yourself because those are the ones that will lift you up or keep you grounded.

Look around you. Think of the people you see. What about those you don't?

Take a deep breath and then close your eyes. Who are the people that quickly come to mind?

Who are those people that teach you, uplift you, and elevate you? Who are the people in your life who helped you along the way? The people you talk to, connect with, interact with, and touch on a daily basis? Stop now. Take a moment and think.

What is it that makes these people so special and so present?

How do these people make you feel? Warm? Happy? Do they make a difference in your life and in the life of others?

Does your heart beat a little faster around them? Does your soul ignite, and do your eyes light up?

Does the world look a little more colorful? Less black and white when they are in your atmosphere?

We repeat: Who are those people that teach you, uplift you, and elevate you? Who are the people in your life who have helped you along the way?

In short, who are your mentors?

Each of our journeys is enriched with influencers. These are the people who served as lighthouses along the way, illuminating the path and ensuring we navigated the rough terrain. As for us, we give enormous credit to our dream team, the group of people that pushes us to do great things. Your influencers could be loved ones, your children, close friends, teachers, coaches, or colleagues.

These people take us under their wings so we can form strong and vibrant wings of our own.

A life without mentors is a less fulfilling life. We all need people to push us hard and expect the best we have within. Life can be challenging, but to know we are not in it alone can often lessen the blows as they come. We relied on a lot of people for their guidance. We navigated oceans of new water, and the endless support we received helped us to make it through with just a few bumps and bruises. Mentors give the gift that keeps on giving. They impart the gifts of time, modeling, advice, and encouragement that can be the difference between succeeding in your dreams or shying away from your opportunities.

So through our experience, we quickly learned that the fourth step in our prescription to create a radical life is to *build a team that supports your dreams.*

We call this our radical Dream Team. We all have those people in our lives that are true difference makers. We can still remember the framed picture of an article our father published for a national journal. He entitled it "You Are My Teachers." He would send us a copy of this article hanging on his wall on what seemed like an annual basis, striving to remind us again and again of the importance of those who came before and those who taught us what we now call our own. For better or worse, the people with whom we surround ourselves will often determine the direction in which we go. And science supports this.

RADICAL *fact*

Glamour magazine reported, "Studies show that women with mentors often earn more than those without."

Women are actively looking for mentors. For example:

One out of five women say they've never had a mentor at work, according to a LinkedIn 2011 survey.

A survey by a women's networking organization, Levo League, found that a whopping 95 percent of women had never sought out a mentor at work.

Caroline Hirons says, "The amount of white middle age men getting awards and running the beauty industry is stunning. We need to promote women in the world of business. Women need to be mentored by women that have walked the road before them."

Think about what this means for each of us. As women, we are simply not using the unbelievable resources that are readily available. And the statistics show that taking advantage of those opportunities mathematically results in greater personal and professional gains. Think about the people in your life for which you carry great respect. Who are they? What do they do? How did they get there?

Caroline continues, "First you have to be open to it. If you know where you want to be and see someone that you want to be like and emulate, go and ask them. Women want to help women. People like to help people. If you tell others that you would like some coaching on how to get where they are, and they say no, then they were not the right mentor to begin with."

Find time to approach those people, schedule a lunch or coffee, and then pick their brains to determine how their experience can assist in your journey.

So it should come as no surprise that to live a radical life, you have to take the steps and actions that others may be unwilling to take. The friends, mentors, colleagues, and team we choose (and it is a choice) will not only support our dreams, they will fast-track them. Radical people surround themselves with radical mentors. And radical mentors help us to live radical lives. It is an exciting proposition that science actually supports encircling your life with people you not only identify with, but who you are also similar to in beliefs, characteristics, and strengths.

Caroline says, "I like the saying that the five people you spend the most time with are a reflection of yourself. Hang out with your people of choice.

Pursue mentors that have the character that you admire. Be discerning with whom you allow in your circle. When someone shows you who they are, believe them. If someone says they are a drunk and cause trouble, believe them. Be careful not to make too many excuses for them."

When we asked Dan Buettner about the importance of mentors and the wisdom they instill, he said, "We live in a society that celebrates youth, and in most of these cultures where people live a long time, they celebrate age. The older you get, the wiser you are. Across the globe, you see examples of mentorship everywhere. On our journey, we met a 102-year-old karate master who was still mentoring people 75 years younger than him. In Okinawa, we met 103-year-old basket weavers teaching 14-year-old girls, passing the traditions down. Mentorship is everywhere."

Your mentors are a strong contributing factor to success. Sometimes you think you're singing to yourself, and all of a sudden you hear a chorus sharing the same tune. You're like, *wow, that's pretty crazy – maybe I'm not alone.* Just the simple fact that you are not alone can oftentimes lift you to where you need to be.

It gave us a lot of support to know that others viewed our business in the same way. Doubt is natural. But you'll find that you have less of it when your Dream Team is rooting you on. So having a team of people you care about acting as your mirror can be a huge deal. Not everyone has mentors readily available. You have to take the time to search them out, ask friends, research relevant topics, and do whatever it takes to surround yourself with the right people. When you begin the process of creating a dream, you'll find that you attract the right type of people into your life. But you need a strong team even before that dream is projected to the world.

RADICAL *thought*

Having a support network of friends is proven to lower stress and improve overall health and well-being.[7]

DREAM ACCELERATORS

We believe that friends, mentors, and colleagues can act as dream accelerators. They can move you in your preferred direction faster than you could on your own. This is attracting alignment. You must be in alignment with the world, with your marketplace, with others, and with yourself.

RADICAL *fact*

When you are out of alignment, you are rarely vibrating at a high level. You are leaving valuable energy and opportunity behind, making it harder to attract your desired outcomes.

Imagine a seesaw. You can't create movement on a seesaw if you are the only one on it. But toss one of your friends on the other side and you will quickly find yourself moving up. The same is true in your journey to live a radical life. If you find mentors with expansive beliefs and qualities, you will move closer to your goals.

Most of us aren't given a whole pie; instead we are given a slice of the pie, and if we can search out others who can help round that out, it will inspire us to be a better version of ourselves, a more fulfilled version, a more impactful version. We should wholeheartedly take those tools and lessons. Everyone is good at something. The more we can learn from the people out there who are crossing in and out of our lives, the better and happier we will be.

Our dear friend Cynthia Kersey, personal coach, motivational speaker, and founder of the Unstoppable Foundation, shared with us an important lesson on the power of sharing what you have. She says, "Through my experiences with cultivating sustainability in developing third-world countries, I have learned some radical lessons. The most important one being that a little bit goes so far. When you provide, it's not a handout; it's a hand-up. We have the opportunity daily to contribute to another's life.

"For example, when I was at a women's conference, I met a girl in her early twenties with a little baby, and I was giving her things. Well, she literally went home and gave it to her family members; she gave it to her friends. It's just the opposite of how we hoard and believe there's not enough; we live from a place of scarcity in such a country of extreme abundance. And they are in extreme poverty, yet when you give them a little bit, they share it."

We can embrace this lesson and share the knowledge we have accumulated with others. Mentors allow us to reach new heights and explore new realms of possibility. If we are all willing to share with each other, just imagine what we can accomplish!

According to *Forbes Magazine, becoming a mentor will also increase your success. Key reasons include: a better understanding of your business, a better understanding of how people perceive you, a larger network, help with solving issues, and personal satisfaction.*

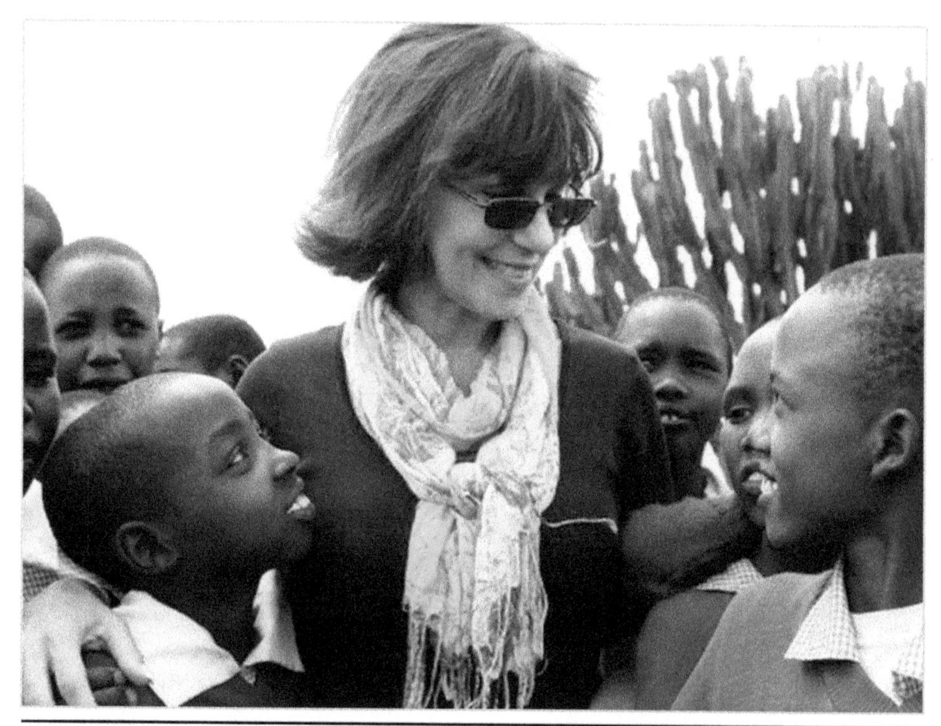

Cynthia Kersey, Unstoppable Foundation, mentoring some of her students, Unstoppablefoundation.org

We never could have reached our goals without strong and supportive mentors.

RADICAL thought

"You've got to find mentors. People will help you if you ask openly. You've got to speak up because if you don't, you'll never know."

Without mentors, we would have been lost. We needed those people who came before us, learned lessons the hard way, and were then willing to share those lessons with us.

Liz: We truly learn from so many people in our life and continue to do so. Therefore, my mentor list grows by the minute. I like to look for and learn from people in the area where I think they represent greatness. I imagine myself as a baby duck, and I find other ducks to look at, to mimic, to walk behind, and say, "Okay, that might not be who I am today, but I want to be like this person. I would like to emulate how this person lives life." I think of myself as a collector of people. I collect amazing people whose light shines on me, and then I carry the light to others.

RADICAL *fact*

Research shows that longevity and happiness are directly related to the community you've created.

We were lucky in so many ways because as sisters we worked together, and we have a great support system between the two of us. Especially when you're growing a business, there is great value in having people surround you who believe in the mission and purpose of what you're going after. Whether you are building a business or building your personal life, a strong friend and a powerful network within your organization focused on that common goal is truly groundbreaking. While we've had experiences of networking with people who aren't completely likeminded, you grow more quickly when you have people who are focused on the same thing and want to reach that goal or that purpose instilled in an organization or in your *life*.

As women, all we have is each other. Yet alarming statistics show that we remain unwilling to work together to mentor one another and reduce the length of the journey for us all. Together we can build a win/win life. Radical living is just that. Through building a radical dream team, you instill a fundamental pillar of support that will always be a welcomed addition to your journey. Our radical prescription pushes you to build your radical dream team and willingly and consciously seek out mentors to help you architect your dream life.

Radical Recap:

When you find yourself searching for Radical Mentors, always remember that:

1. Mentors empower. Assemble your team of radical mentors early and rely upon them often.

2. Each of our journeys is enriched with influencers. These are the people who served as lighthouses along the way, illuminating the path to help us navigate through the rough terrain. Find your lighthouse.

3. Mentors are everywhere. There is no perfect recipe to find those that can help you along the way. Listen with open ears to ensure that you find your teammates.

4. It is an honor to be asked to be a mentor and share your knowledge and guidance. Both people receive a gift in that relationship. Be fearless and simply ask or offer to help another.

5. Women like to help women and people like to help people. Surround yourself with people that reflect the you that you want to be.

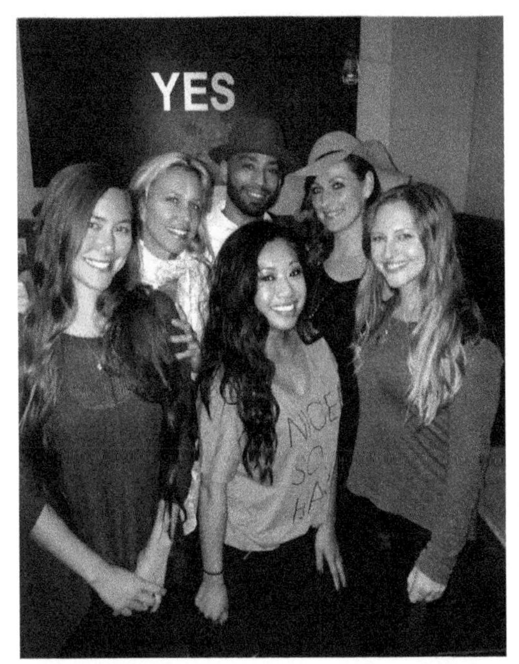
YES

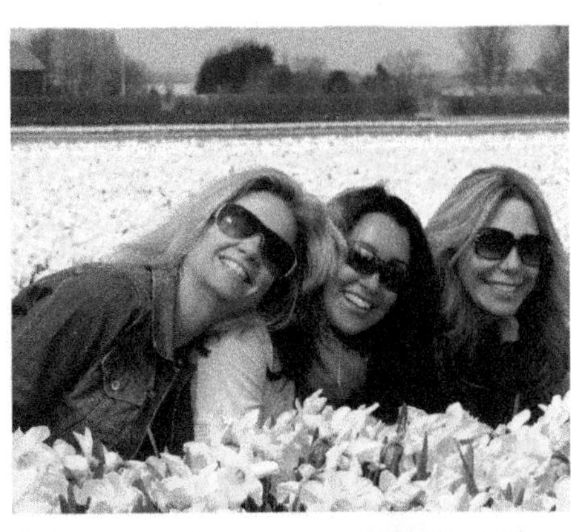

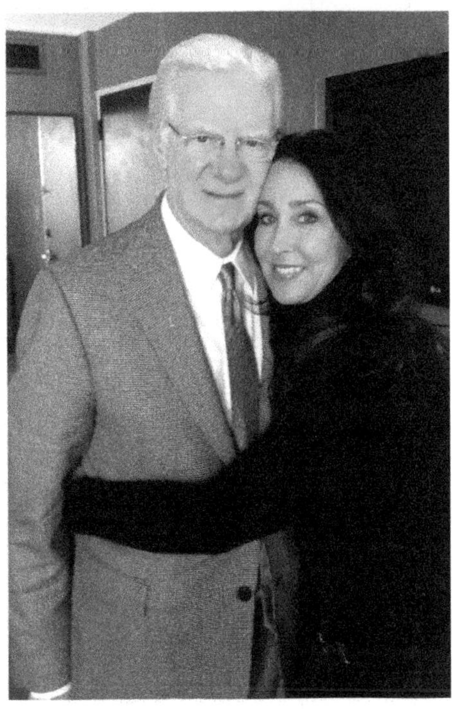

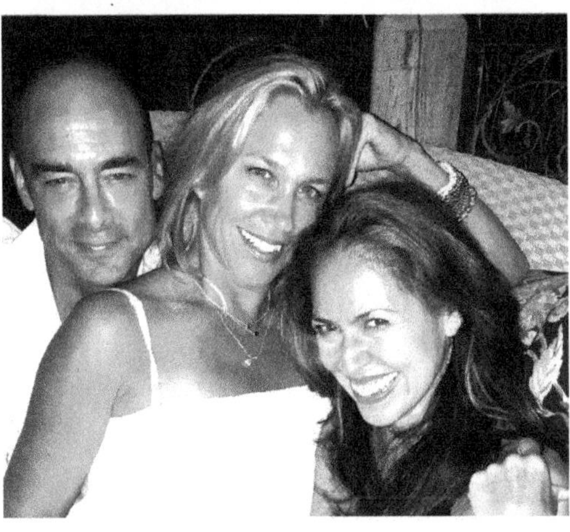

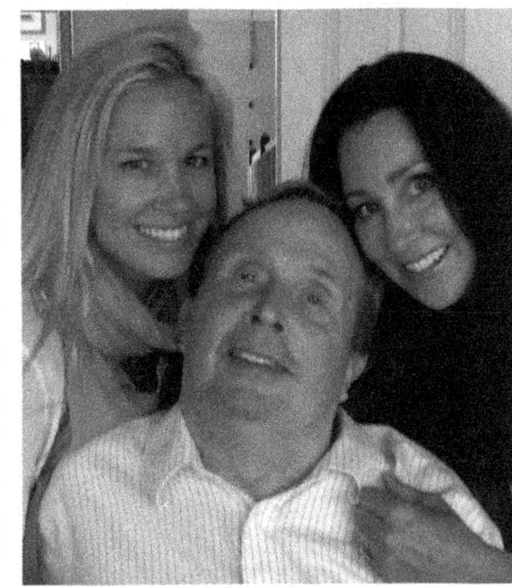

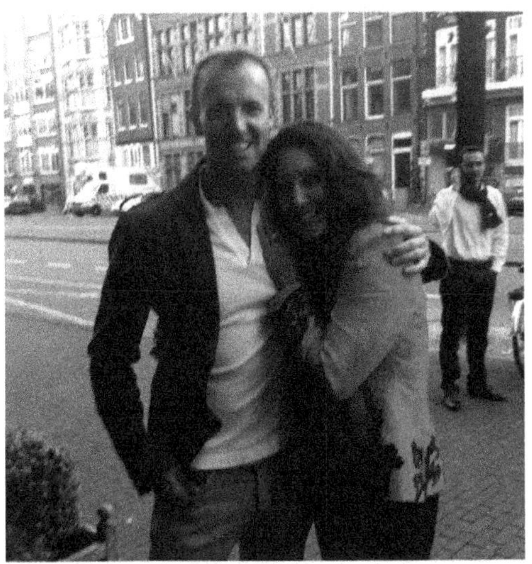

Chapter 11:
RADICAL DIFFERENCE

There are over seven billion people in the world.

Think of the possibilities when half of the world's population strives to make one bit of difference in the life of another.

That would mean that 3.5 billion lives would be improved.

Even if it is something as small as a compliment?

Consider what the world would look like with 3.5 billion more smiles each day!

Well, the simple math would show that our world would be inundated with 105 billion more smiles each month, and 1.2 trillion more smiles each year. We would find it hard for anyone to argue that 1.2 trillion more smiles wouldn't be a difference maker in the world.

Scientists have proven that the average child laughs 300 times a day, while the average adult only laughs six to eight times each day. You have to wonder, where did the other 290-plus laughs go?

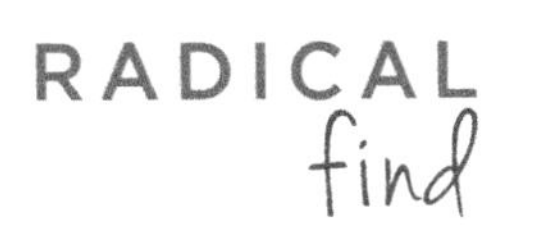

Research shows that smiling is in fact contagious! It is hard to frown when looking at someone else's smile. It also helps boost your immune system by aiding in relaxation.[9]

Mahatma Gandhi said, "Be the difference you want to see in the world."

For us, living a radical life means helping others live radical lives. Remember, your mentors and friends are those folks that help you get off the ground. And in turn, you have the radical responsibility to do the same for another. Imagine how truly amazing the world would be if we each decided to spend just a few minutes every day making a difference in the life of even one person.

We were lucky. Our father, mother, and friends were our Gandhi. Our dad always reminded us that to make a difference you have to *be* the difference. On a daily basis, our mother would constantly ask us what action we took to make a difference in the life of another. Not all of us had this mentorship, but with a little conscious effort (which for sure you have), you are the difference and can project that to the world.

When we started Radical Skincare, we did so to solve a personal problem. Eventually we found a higher calling. As we saw how many smiles our regimen improved, we found that we could make a difference in the lives of people across the world. By playing a small yet humble role in making people feel more confident in their appearance, we helped them to be more present in their lives, more comfortable in their skin, and more able to make a difference in the lives of others. Taking a life-changing skincare line and deciding to share it with people across the globe was not easy. But we felt strongly that we could change skin and then change lives.

Rachel: My condition was unbearable. I was embarrassed and didn't even recognize myself. And I knew millions of people across the world experienced the same condition. So when Radical Skincare made a difference in my life, I knew pretty quickly it could make a difference in the lives of others. So we accepted the opportunity to be difference makers and reached out to our dream team, those mentors who could shed light on a path we had not traveled and give us directions and landmarks to look for so that we could embark upon a radical journey of our own.

Becoming a difference maker is an important step in the prescription for a radical life because it is the culmination of everything that came before. You can't work to change the lives of others unless you first change your own life. For us, we underwent a substantial journey through radical living. And only when we felt our lives were radical did we think about sharing it with the world. But we quickly learned that the difference is in the details.

My vision is that we will have touched enough people in an organic way that they will look through the radical lens at their world with the belief that anything is possible. If I am remembered as a person who gave a human and honest element to an industry that has been skin-deep, or as a person who showed that the simple moments of going above and beyond can better your life and the lives of others, I will have accomplished something worthwhile. I think about it often and try to imagine what people will say when I am gone.

I want to know that my work impacts others and helps people achieve their dreams. This means a lot to me. It is truly an inside-out approach. Being a mother who helps guide my kids to develop into unique individuals is important for me. Also, being remembered as a great friend, wife, mentor and mother is a dream of mine.

Why does radical empowerment and making a difference matter to you? It matters because it is part of your legacy. One impactful exercise is to imagine your funeral and what people would say about you. What would be written on a tombstone or in your obituary? What would people say at your funeral about you?

What do you do to impact another's life?

What would people write in your obituary?

Why not write your own today and spend tomorrow living the person that you want to be?

T. Harv Eker said, "How you do anything is how you do everything." We think that this has a lot of truth to it. Today we work to focus on being a difference. We are clearly not alone. We are among the groundswell of people who have noticed that the power of giving is one of the keys to riches and happiness.

RADICAL *fact*

According to the National Philanthropic Trust, 95.4 percent of households give to charity with an annual household contribution of $2,974.

But it gets better...

In 2013 alone, Americans gave $335.17 billion to charity. And individuals were the largest source of charitable giving at $241.32 billion, or 72 percent of total giving, followed by foundations ($50.28 billion or 15 percent), bequests ($26.81 billion or 8 percent), and corporations ($16.76 billion or

5 percent). These numbers are staggering. And they support the point that we as humans *want* to make a difference. We are not only wired to do so, we actively do so.

So much of this is accomplished through compassion and care for others. Not everyone is as fortunate as we are. Many people need our help. They need the difference makers. Radical people are difference makers. They not only search for the need, they work to fulfill it.

Compassion, care, and helping others, are the underpinnings that move people to help others.

In fact, science supports this very notion. "Recipients of kindness generally want to keep paying it forward," says James Fowler, professor of medical genetics and political science at the University of California, San Diego. In one of Fowler's studies, he found that a single act of kindness typically inspired several more acts of generosity. The scientific name for this chain of altruism is "upstream reciprocity," but you can think of it as a domino effect of warm and fuzzy feelings. If you drop a quarter into an expired parking meter, the recipient of that small act of generosity will be inspired to do a kind act for someone else, and on and on.

Similarly, our Uncle Ted has always inspired us with his ability to make a difference. Growing up, he was Uncle Ted the Giant Crab, who would chase us around on the floor and tickle us until we would literally say *"Uncle!"*

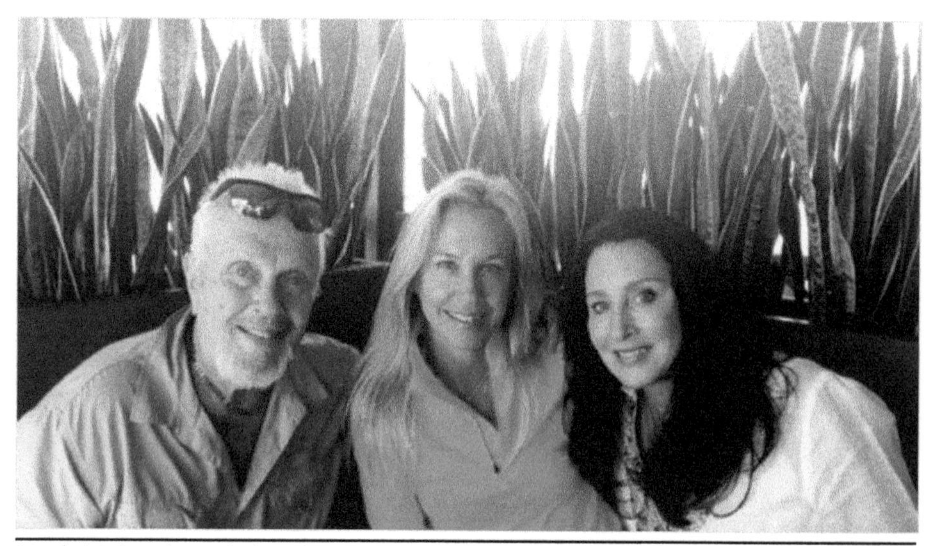

Uncle Ted with Rachel and Liz

As we grew as women, we realized that Uncle Ted had the same radical roots that underpinned who and what we are today. When we spoke, he told us of how Total Action Against Poverty helped to find a solution for medical care in low-income regions.

He said, "We decided to help find a solution to the issue of medical care. In the impoverished parts of our state, children were getting sicker and sicker because they were not receiving proper healthcare. So we gathered the local physicians to determine why this occurred. What we found was that children were not receiving healthcare because they could not get rides to their appointments. We always thought it was an issue of payment, but it really was an issue of access. Many times these children and their families didn't make their appointments or weren't able to follow through. They didn't get to their medication. And when they did not make their appointments, thousands of dollars in Medicaid would be wasted and doctors would have a gap in their schedule. It was literally a whole bunch of wasted resources. And so we created a program that provided family advocacy to utilize the medical system and actually show up for the pre-paid appointments. To date, this program has been in effect for over twenty years and has served over fifteen hundred children. It has been a successful project ensuring that these children get excellent healthcare, and a good, healthy start in life."

Anything is possible when people identify the root of the problem and go beneath the surface to understand the real issues at hand. The magic comes when we work together to support one another. We are all difference makers. Both science and statistics support this notion. We simply cannot do it alone.

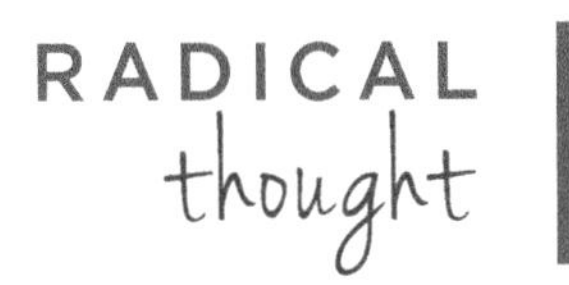

The prescription for living a radical life calls for you to be the difference. And to remember that the small differences are oftentimes the most important ones.

Living a radical life is at our fingertips.

Karl Marx said, "To be radical is to grasp things by the root." We have discussed our roots at length. We are a product of our mentors, of saying yes, and of looking toward the opportunity in adversity. A radical prescription is easy to follow. It is a series of shifts that will reward you with unbelievable movement. You are radical at your root and at your core. It is all about uncovering it, discovering it, and expressing it. Once you shift your lens to do this, a world of opportunity awaits you and is yours for the taking.

Everyone has radical DNA. The stories we want to share are life moments that we all have that can inspire others. The question we all must ask is how can we make an impact, either big or small? How can we grow and make our world a better place?

You can be the difference.

Uncle Ted said, "I think radical is seeing how you could really make a difference in the lives of other people. You could do it on a one-to-one basis or work to actually change the systems and modify them so that people have a greater opportunity. There is a lot of pressure to maintain the status quo. But once you start asking questions you can begin the process of changing the systems that might not be working so well. Now that's radical. For me, I'm just a persistent, sometimes obnoxious son of a bitch that keeps pushing the envelope and isn't scared of throwing some elbows from time to time. That has been my way of doing things."

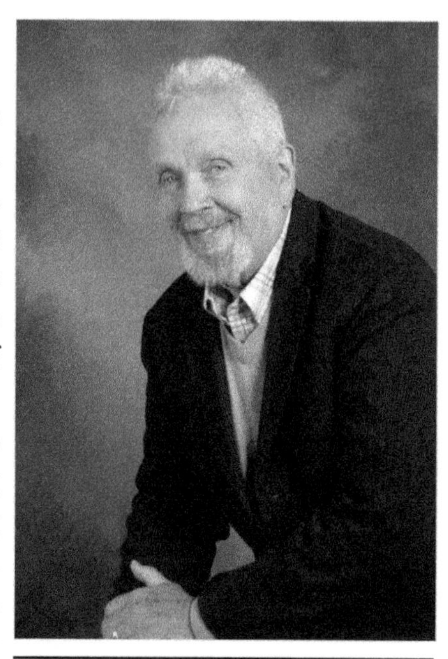

Author and Nonprofit Advocate Ted Edlich

MAKING A DIFFERENCE

The big things and the little things count; all things count. That is who we are and what we are about, and that is who you are. Radical DNA is coursing through your veins just waiting to be expressed. As we walk through our lives we are constantly amazed at the opportunities before us to make the radical difference for another and inevitably for ourselves. Giving is getting. It is the law of the universe. You just need to listen and hear the possibilities that are there for you to exercise your giving muscle.

Possibilities are plentiful, and the brilliant part of it is that the better you get at it, the better your life and the more fulfillment you will enjoy. What good are your assets unless you share them? Assets are not just money assets or material things; they can also be a talent or strength you use to help another. We all have an abundance of life assets. It may be a social network you have that can help another, and the list goes on.

Liz: One moment to make a difference and empower another to pursue their dreams occurred as I was relaxing at our home in Little Exuma, Bahamas. Living on an island in the Bahamas had been a goal and dream of mine since I was a teenager, and I also had written down the goal of living on an island numerous times as it truly was one of my heart's desires. Given the power of visualization and goal setting, it is no wonder I ended up with a home there to enjoy for the last seventeen years.

Gloria, Miss Glo, as we call her, a Jamaican woman who lives on the property and takes care of our home, had her grandson Chaddy staying with her for a couple of months over the summer. This was the second time that I had met him.

He was soft-spoken and spent quite a bit of time to himself. I asked Chaddy and Miss Glo to join us for dinner in hopes of getting to know him better. As we discussed his life in Jamaica, I learned that he was in line to be a police officer. A police officer in Jamaica sounded like a death sentence to me, and as mild-mannered as he was, it also seemed an odd choice.

Come to find out later in the conversation, it wasn't his first choice or desire at all. It was the only choice available because if one didn't have the money to continue a higher education, that was his only path to income.

I asked Chaddy if he had a passion or a dream of what he wanted, and he immediately responded that drawing was his passion and that his dream was to be an architect, but he could not afford the $2750 tuition. He said with a twinkle in his eye that drawing was his life and then promptly showed me some of the sketches he did of different people that were a shockingly good resemblance. He also explained that he had learned to draw on his own and had never had any formal training. It was evident he was a gifted young man.

I asked Chaddy if he wanted to work to earn his tuition, and he explained that he had applied numerous places in vain due to the high unemployment rate in Jamaica. I asked how many more days he was staying at our Sugar Beach Villa home, and he said twenty-seven more days before his return to Jamaica.

I was curious as to how badly he really wanted his tuition, as I have watched many kids in this generation say they truly desire something, but they do not have the persistence and fortitude to work for it and do whatever it takes to get there. At times, we as parents assist in this, paving the way for our children and thereby making it far too easy for them to get what they want. Many times this deprives them of the joy of seeing the fruits of their labor to create an outcome that leads to success and opportunity. I believe these are important building blocks that build self-sufficiency and a belief that you can do what it takes, no matter what.

Fortunately, Chaddy was up for the challenge and took me up on my offer to work. The job was not an easy one. He needed to clear out the dense bush areas on the property for fifteen dollars an hour for the next twenty-seven days. At the end of the month he could return to Jamaica and register for university and pursue his dream.

Eight o'clock the next morning, with the temperature already at 80 degrees, I heard the hatchet and sickle in the bush. I walked down to say good morning and bring Chaddy some water. I told him I was going be away for the day but I would love for him to join us for dinner again.

Every day of my holiday I woke to the sound of chopping and raking in the bush. A big smile would grace his lips as we would *oooh* and *ahh* at his remarkable and artistic progress. He did more in the seven days that I was there than I ever witnessed anyone do in our seventeen years of living there.

It was a terrific win/win; Chaddy was working to pay for his dream and I was getting a beautiful landscaping job. I could have given him the money and "sponsored" him as they call it in the Bahamas. But I did not want to rob him of the gift of feeling accomplished. Something happens when you are able to experience and to witness the result of what you committed to and it paid off. It is a sweet dessert and provides learning and conditioning that can be carried over to other areas of work, play, sports, fitness, health, and relationships. It builds a sense of drive to achieve the reward of accomplishment and success.

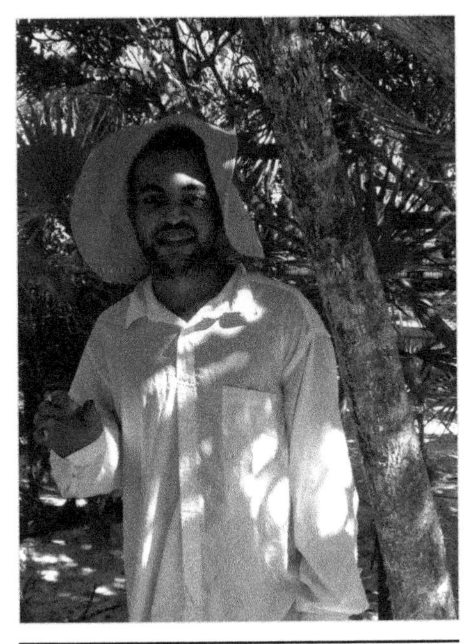

Chaddy at work

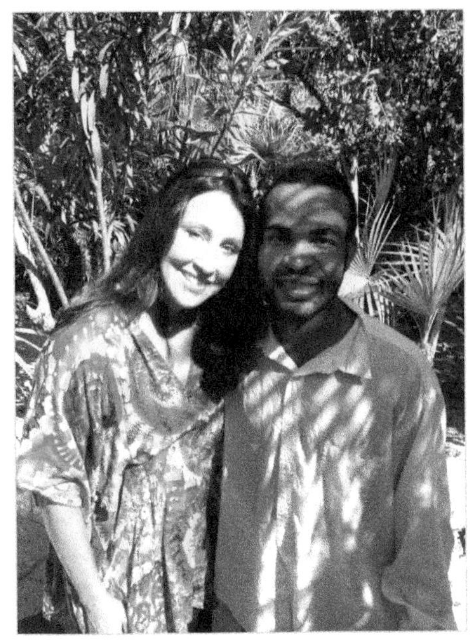

Liz/Chaddy together

Before the publishing of this book, I sent Chaddy this story. He responded to me and said, "Miss Liz- thank you so much. You mean so much to me and if there weren't a you, then I wouldn't be pursuing my goals now. Sometimes I sit down and look back on life and my eyes full with tears to see how hard it was for me. But God always works in mysterious ways and I believe you are the angel that he sent for me. Thank you so much."

In my case, the radical opportunity to empower another's dreams, and use my assets to support this well-deserving young man, was a real gift to me. My days became more purposeful as I watched this young man work toward what he wanted, saw the pride in his grandmother's face, and realized that for years to come the cleared and sculpted garden that I would walk through would be a sweet reminder of Chaddy's journey of pursuing his dream and giving me the opportunity to empower him and be a small part of his quest.

RADICAL EMPOWERMENT

When we speak about being radical, it's about tapping into our DNA and seeing the opportunities to go above and beyond to make a difference.

The act of empowering another is a gift that we all can give.

Feeling empowered is typically learned, earned, or supported.

When we empower another in a situation where they may not feel able, it is an opportunity to ignite the gifts we were given and use them to better another. Many times the magic in life lives in its simplicity, and therefore the ability to empower or support another is in front of you on a daily basis – often in the simplest of moments.

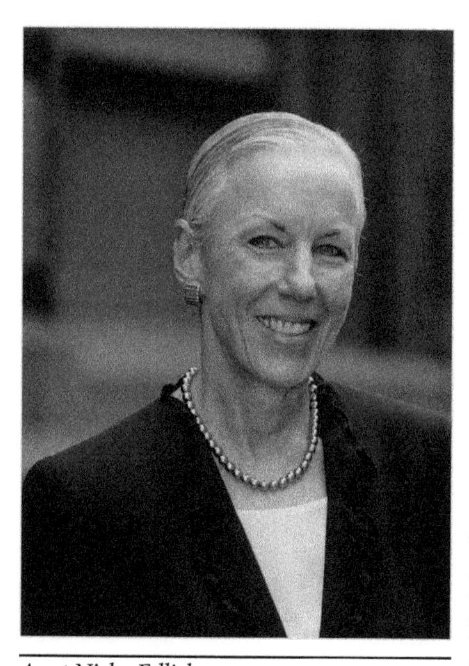

Aunt Nicky Edlich

Before Aunt Nicky passed, we went to dinner in NYC with her and Aunt Karen. We call them "the Aunties." Aunt Nicky had been battling cancer for over nine years and had most recently entered into new programs of exotic chemo cocktails that made her feel ill and weak.

Her fortitude was compelling in her effort to capture life and embrace every precious moment. The price she was willing to pay is significant but worth it, as she would say. It's that way with anything worth fighting for, and life for sure is one of those things.

Radical empowerment gives us the opportunity to stand for something greater than ourselves and to fight for another who might not be as capable, strong at the moment, or willing. Standing for another when they are not able to fight for themselves at that moment is a radical opportunity to make a difference.

Our Aunt Nicky did this in one of her last chemo sessions as she sat in the waiting room with an older Asian woman waiting for their respective treatments. As they waited for close to an hour in an environment that is fraught with harsh reality and reminders of how precious one's health and life is, the nurse arrived and spoke to the lady next to her and proceeded to give her a slip telling her that it wasn't possible to see her because they were backed up. The slip had a date and time on it suggesting that she return in two days for treatment. When fighting for your life, you would hope that the mismanagement of a treatment center would not add to the struggle and threaten your treatment.

The older woman did not respond much, and our aunt leaned over and asked, "Excuse me, did you understand what she said?" The woman nodded and said in broken English that she understood she had to come back another day. Aunt Nicky then asked, "How long did it take you to get here?" The woman replied that she lived in the Brooklyn and that it took her well over an hour because she had to take three trains to get there.

Aunt Nicky's sense of injustice was growing by the minute and she decided to take a radical stand to empower this woman to get the treatment she deserved and to challenge the system.

She called over the attendant and explained the situation. The attendant not surprisingly said that was the way it was. Aunt Nicky insisted that she speak to a supervisor. She insisted that it was not okay to make an elderly woman make this type of travel in the heat of summer, by train, when she had an appointment, and at the very least they should hire transportation to drive her home and bring her back on the day of her new appointment.

After challenging the system, Aunt Nicky prevailed and her newfound friend was escorted upstairs for her treatment.

To put this into perspective, think for just a moment about the absolute rage you have probably witnessed with young, able, and healthy people when their flight is delayed in an airport. This woman traveled to save or extend her life, barely speaks English, and because of her language barrier, age, culture, or personality, is in a position that, if unchecked, would have resulted in the thoughtless dismissal of her chemo session.

As we listened to this story we were moved to tears, seeing our aunt with her own burden, a person with a life-threatening illness that eventually took her from us, going out of her way to care for a stranger in a waiting room because she could, and it made a difference. It's what a road less traveled can look like in real everyday life.

For one thing it can be unpopular; you can only imagine how many of the staff considered our aunt a "pain in the ass" that day. But doesn't it make sense to challenge a situation that we know doesn't support a person, even if it is unpopular?

It brought us back to our father and mother and the philosophy that was front and center in our household growing up.

Our philosophy is one to fight for the underdog, the one who is less able, to support the weakling in school, stand against religious or ethnic prejudice, and to give to those in need because you are able. Our parents walked the talk and provided us with a great example to remember and carry on. Get behind what you believe.

Caroline Hirons shares, "People many times say that I am opinionated. I am not necessarily opinionated, I simply voice my opinion. I believe that you have to speak your mind and voice your mind. You are entitled to. Don't be afraid to say what you think, what you feel, and what you need. Don't tolerate things. Women tolerate so much. If it feels wrong, say its wrong. If in your gut it feels wrong, then say it. Your intuition is probably spot on."

She continues, "We never know how what we do or say can make a difference in the life of another. I was doing a personal appearance and a woman came up to me and said you saved my life. She said that she was in a domestic violence situation and was going to kill herself. She was lying in bed with the pills all lined up and ready to swallow them to once and for all to put an end to her pain. She was on Twitter and watched one of my videos. Then she started reading my blog. She said that my message was so empowering that 5 hours later she was still reading and watching. Suddenly, she realized that she didn't want to kill herself anymore. Today she is in a new relationship and the court case of the abuse she suffered is coming up. She took a page out of my message of empowerment to speak out and honor herself. We never know how what we are doing will touch and change the course of another."

It is important to model these types of behaviors for our children and contribute to a collective consciousness that empowers others and makes a difference.

Think about it: you, a loved one, or your child goes into a hospital for treatment and because it saves the hospital money, you are exposed to something life threatening like powdered latex gloves? What consumer spends time studying the gloves that a doctor uses to operate, a dentist uses in their mouth, etc.? We venture to guess, very few. So isn't it incumbent upon us, if we know a better way, to take a stand for what we know makes a difference? From his wheelchair, our father wrote a book, *Medicine's Deadly Dust* and petitioned the FDA to remove powdered gloves from the market. The ban was finally granted the week before he died.

Whether sitting in a chemo waiting room, having the knowledge of a better and more healthy way to treat others in medicine, or standing up in the most simple of situations for those less able – the elderly, a child, an animal—it is all an opportunity to tap into the radical DNA that is within all of us. It gives us daily the opportunity to craft our eulogy with a storyline we are proud of. Get radical and empower others, because you can and it makes a difference

One of our favorite stories goes as follows: A little girl is walking down the beach and sees that the beach is littered with thousands of starfish washed up on the sand. Further down the beach she notices an older man picking up the starfish one by one and throwing them back into the water. Eager to understand the method behind this madness, she runs up and asks, "What are you doing?" "I am picking up the starfish and throwing them back into the ocean or they will die," he replies. To that she stares puzzled and then looks further down the beach and sees miles of starfish before her. She says, "Mister, there are thousands of starfish on this beach; do you really think that you can make a difference?" The old man picks up a starfish, shows it to her, and says, "To this one it makes a difference," and with that he throws the starfish back into the ocean and continues on his journey.

Let the lens that you peer through be radical and make a difference.

Radical Recap:

To work towards making a radical difference, always remember that:

1. Living a radical life is at our fingertips. We can accomplish this by becoming a difference maker in the world.
2. It is the little things and the big things. It does not take much to make a difference. Often times, love, attention, and a little bit of your time and energy does the trick.
3. Be Radical and get behind what you believe. A little bit of passion and purpose can go a long way in making a difference.
4. Empower another to see their greatness.
5. Stand up for yourself and others. Stand for what you know can make a difference.
6. Your legacy is written daily in how you show up to create a life worth loving.

Chapter 12:
RADICAL BELIEF

Belief is one of the most powerful cornerstones of living a life you love.

And it is a crucial part of our prescription for living a radical life.

Belief in your innate ability to do what needs to be done.

Belief in yourself. Belief that anything is possible.

Belief is the lubrication for success, and when it comes to creating a radical life, if you believe it then you can achieve it.

If you believe something will work, it often can. However, if you believe it won't work, it never really had a chance in the first place. American philosopher William James said, "Believe that life is worth living and your belief will help create the fact." A radical life starts with a radical belief system, one that is dedicated to the cause and to the notion that you can get it done. With this in mind, think of the possibilities.

Think of giving a troubled young child a pill and telling him he will find himself happy, centered, and more successful than ever before if he just takes that pill for a month.

What if he believed you?

What if you gave a college student a pill and told him it would help him to get straight A's?

What if he actually believed you?

What if you gave a man in an unhappy marriage a pill and told him it would help him find the love he lost for his wife?

What if he actually believed you?

A paradigm is a pattern or a way in which you view your life. Bob Proctor often speaks of paradigms. He indicates that paradigms are simply conditioned habits created as early as childhood that live in our subconscious mind. Oftentimes the results we obtain have very little to do with the knowledge we have. We know there is a fast lane to get us to our desired goal. We just don't actually make the lane change to get onto that highway because our conditioning tells us the lane is full or not for us. But our current conditioning is the real reason we remain in a slow lane making little progress while cars pass us by. In all actuality, those that raised us and surround us actually program our lifestyle and behavior.

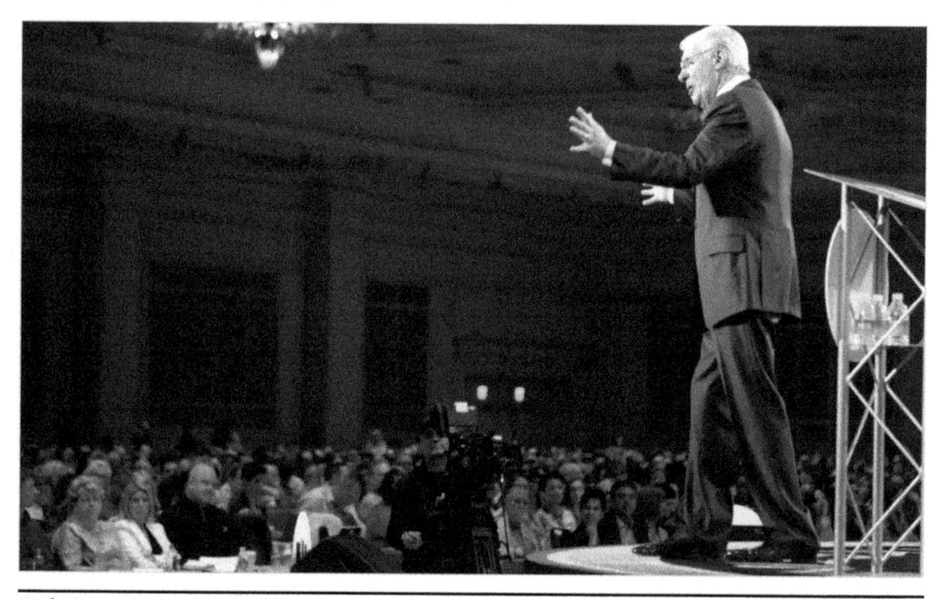

Bob Proctor at one of his seminars speaking to an engaged audience

For more about Bob Proctor's story visit his Living Portrait on the Radical Living section of our website www.radicalskincare.com/living.

Our conscious mind is where our intellect resides. But our behavior is controlled by our subconscious mind, which is the location of this ever-powerful paradigm.

Our paradigms and limiting beliefs are very influential. We either tend to see them and accept them, or not see them at all and just endure them "as the way things are and always will be." We are powerless to them if we do not recognize them and then expose them in order to challenge their veracity.

So the best defense is knowledge. Take the time to write down your beliefs. Most times, you'll find that you inherited these beliefs. We all maintain the ability to shift paradigms and to change our lives. There is a program in our mind that controls our life. As we change our paradigms and subconscious habits, our beliefs begin to shift. And as we write our own paradigm and take control of our lives, we have the opportunity and ability to live in the way we so desire. But it all starts with that shift in our subconscious belief system and obtaining the knowledge that these limiting beliefs are even there.

Lavinia Errico reminds us, "Radical belief means you believe something with your whole self. You don't just use words. The 'language' isn't enough. You have to do the work. You have to do it to see that it works, and then you can believe. You have to take the journey toward belief." When we take the journey to radical belief, we open ourselves to self-growth, which in turn increases our chances for success.

What if we lived in a world where imagination and belief could truly manifest that which you visualize and dedicate yourself to, even if it was scientifically and logically inexplicable? The truth is that we do. There are thousands of examples of how belief has overcome all odds and disproved anything and everything in its path. Radical belief can manifest unbelievably radical results. But you have to first dedicate yourself and truly buy in, placebo or otherwise.

Our friend Roger Linse says, "Believe in the unbelievable to make the impossible possible." For years we lived by a similar credo and said, "Fake it till you make it." At the core of both of these life mantras is believing in yourself and something bigger than yourself. Regardless of your circumstances, if you believe it, then you can achieve it. While the belief to achieve may sound trite and overused, it is actually quite direct and the point of the exercise. Without belief, it is very difficult to persevere and achieve your ultimate dreams.

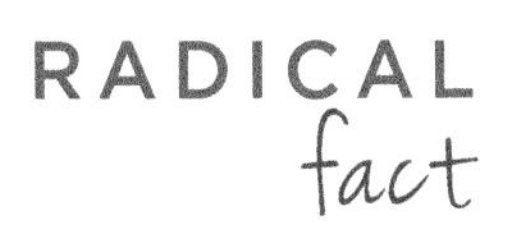

"Fake it till you make it" may have scientific support; psychologists posit that making yourself smile can reverse a bad mood![10]

Personally, we believe that living a radical life calls for a steadfast and impactful belief system that *you* design and adopt. Eventually it becomes the unwavering guiding light that illuminates your path. It elevates, uplifts, and propels you forward. Think of belief as the gas in your engine. You control the accelerator, and the more you put the pedal to the metal to empower these beliefs, the faster you get where you want to go.

We were lucky. Our parents worked hard to instill in us an enormously strong belief system that anything was possible and that we could make a difference. They told us we could be anything we wanted to be. That was a consistent message throughout our lives.

Dad used to say: "You can be the president of the United States one day."

Our response: "But I don't want that job, Daddy."

Whether or not he suggested the job of our dreams, he voiced a belief that inspired big thinking and opened our minds to a world of unlimited possibility.

It helped to lay the foundation for our radical life to come. Our parents planted the seeds for our radical belief system at a young age, which subscribed to the notion of limitless opportunity, and reminded us that there are literally no boundaries to where we can go. The reality is that both of our parents had to overcome huge obstacles to achieve the life they were living, and their belief that the impossible was possible propelled them to overcome and conquer.

They lived it and we saw it.

Your belief is the core of how you see yourself. It's a strong cord that runs through the fabric of people and is a combination of how you view the world, how you see yourself, and what you choose. Your belief system is your choice.

BELIEF IS...

How we define belief is one thing; how we act upon our belief is something entirely different. The old saying goes, "Actions speak louder than words." When it comes to belief, that couldn't be more accurate. So for our radical conversation, we define belief to be something a little different from what you might expect.

- *Radical belief is a choice*
- *Radical belief changes your mind to change your life*
- *Radical belief is committed conviction*

Radical Belief Is a Choice...

Knowing that belief is a choice will help to create what it is you want. Sometimes there is a clear path. The lights are on or the torch is in your hand. You can clearly see in front of you. Maintaining belief during a time of absolute clarity is easier than when the path ahead is dark and keeping the lights on isn't easy. As you journey through your life, at times the lights may dim or temporarily burn out. The radical challenge is maintaining faith in your belief when the lights are out.

RADICAL *fact*

Renowned research scientist Dr. Bruce H. Lipton believes that our DNA responds to signals from outside our cells, meaning it responds to the energy created by our positive and negative thoughts. His book The Biology of Belief explores and explains these findings in great detail.[11]

Richard Ruffalo, master motivator, author, educator, and internationally recognized athlete, inspires a wide range of audiences everywhere. From children to adults to students to business gurus, Ruffalo is a true role model for all ages. At age thirty-two, Ruffalo lost his eyesight but never lost his "vision." He was diagnosed with a rare degenerative eye disease that gradually made him go blind.

At the Walt Disney McDonald's American Teacher Awards, Ruffalo was named both the Outstanding Coach of the Year and the Outstanding Teacher of the Year for 1995. As a favored citizen of Belleville, New Jersey, he received the "Outstanding Citizen of the Year" award in 1994. He is the winner of four different world titles in shot put, discus, javelin, and powerlifting. He has earned fourteen international gold medals, won thirty-two national titles, set nine world records, and fifteen national records.

And he did all of this after his "lights went out" and he could no longer see. He says, "The secret of success as we journey through our book of life is never to stop when adversity strikes, but simply to keep turning the pages because a better chapter lies ahead." A clear way to deal with loss of external vision is to have a strong inner vision.

RADICAL *thought*

Remember that when the lights go out, your belief can act as your vision, but only if you make that choice.

Rich Ruffalo borrowed the vision of others at first. But then he developed his own clear and lucid vision. He made a choice that even though his lights went out, he would still see all that was ahead of him. It grew from faith and an unshakable belief that he could see with his faith even after his vision was gone.

RADICAL BELIEF CHANGES YOUR MIND TO CHANGE YOUR LIFE...

Radical belief is powerful. But it is also empowering. Our close friend Bob Proctor always says to us, "When you are faced with difficult times, the facts don't matter. Facts always change. When your belief in something is so strong, it can override the facts and the circumstances that appear before you. This is a very powerful tool and will give you an edge in the world." When you believe something, you tend to see the world through that lens that will call in and attract things that support your belief. You can't imagine how often we have to repeat this to ourselves when doubt creeps in. The facts don't matter, they always change. Change is inevitable.

There is scientific evidence that radical belief can truly change your world and your life.

Consider the placebo effect. A placebo is a fake treatment that can sometimes improve a patient's condition simply because the person has the expectation that it will be helpful. Take a second and think about what that means. Medicine is powerful. It cures, it heals, and it can completely change the environment of an individual's overall health. But the placebo effect stands for the proposition that there is no greater or more powerful medicine than that of an individual's belief system. Belief can literally cure all. For example, consider the true story of David Seidler, winner of an Oscar for his original screenplay and major motion picture *The King's Speech.*

His story starts with the question: *Can you imagine cancer away?*

Seidler says he visualized his cancer away. "I know it sounds awfully Southern California and woo-woo, but that's what happened," he admits when he describes the visualization techniques he used when his bladder cancer was diagnosed nearly six years ago.

"When I was first diagnosed in 2005, I was rather upset, of course," Seidler says in a telephone interview from his home in Malibu, California. "After three to four days of producing a lot of mucus and salty tears, I knew prolonged grief was bad for the autoimmune system, and the autoimmune system was the only buddy I had in fighting cancer."

Seidler said that's when he decided to sit down and write the screenplay for *The King's Speech,* which had been simmering in his brain for many years. "I thought, if I throw myself into the creative process, I can't be sitting around feeling sorry for myself," he says.

After consulting with California urologist Dr. Dino DeConcini, Seidler decided not to have chemotherapy or have all or part of his bladder removed, common treatments for bladder cancer. Instead, he opted for surgery to remove just the cancer itself, and he took supplements meant to enhance his immune system. "For years, whenever I walked down the stairs I rattled like a pair of maracas, I had so many pills in me," he says.

But even then, he was unhappy with his condition. And despite his efforts, his cancer returned months later. As his doctor booked an appointment for surgery two weeks later, Seidler commiserated with his soon-to-be ex-wife, and it was a comment from her that gave him the idea to try to visualize his cancer disappearing. "She said, 'Well, what happens if in two weeks they go in and there's no cancer?' I thought to myself that's the dumbest thing I've ever heard. This woman's in total denial."

So Seidler began thinking and visualizing. "I spent hours visualizing a nice, cream-colored unblemished bladder lining, and then I went in for the operation, and a week later the doctor called me and his voice was very strange," Seidler remembers. "He said, 'I don't know how to explain it, but there's no cancer there.'" He says the doctor was so confounded he sent the tissue from the pre-surgical biopsy to four different labs, and all confirmed they were non-cancerous.

Seidler says the doctor couldn't explain how it had happened. But Seidler could. He says he believes the supplements and visualizations were behind what his doctor called a "spontaneous remission" – plus a change in his way of thinking. He stopped feeling sorry for himself because of his cancer. And lo and behold, it cured his cancer.

Dr. Christiane Northrup, a best-selling author who's written extensively on the mind-body connection, says, "This doesn't sound woo-woo to me. The mind has the power to heal." As CNN reports, in research done by the Yale School of Public Health and the National Institute of Aging, young people who had positive perceptions about aging were less likely to have a heart attack or stroke when they grew older. In another study by researchers at Yale and Miami University, middle-aged and elderly people lived seven years longer if they had a positive perception about aging.

Even the American Cancer Society recognizes and pays attention to the placebo effect. On their website, they say, "Even though they don't act on the disease, placebos seem to affect how people feel. This happens in up to 1 out of 3 people." The point of this section is not to argue that the placebo effect is real, but rather to show scientific and real proof that there is nothing more powerful than belief.

RADICAL BELIEF IS COMMITTED CONVICTION...

Radical belief isn't always popular. In fact, it can often be viewed as a slightly against-the-grain, buck-the-trends, and forget-the-odds type of life. Radical belief is the type of belief that isn't always celebrated at first, but often, in hindsight, is truly remarkable. Throughout history, trailblazers and pioneers have come along with remarkably radical beliefs.

In fact, their beliefs have become their calling cards and mission statements, inscribing them in our history books, but more importantly, leaving a lasting impact that has truly changed the world. Most of these radical believers can be defined by just one word. It was the word that drove them to action when others were unwilling to act. And it all started with their desire and inner fire that burned so hot they simply could not extinguish it.

Here are just a few examples of radical believers committed to conviction:

- *Martin Luther King Jr. = Equality*
- *Susan B. Anthony = Temperance*
- *Walt Disney = Imagination*
- *Rosa Parks = Desegregation*
- *Charles Darwin = Evolution*
- *Helen Keller = Education*
- *Albert Einstein = Thought*
- *Amelia Earhart = Flight*

The list goes on and on. Each of these radical individuals was willing to stand where others would not and subscribe to a belief system that transcended the norm because the norm wasn't all that normal. From today's perspective, it is almost unthinkable to consider that we once lived in a segregated and unequal world where imagination didn't exist and we were constrained by the people who ran the world. But for the people mentioned above, we never would have evolved and would remain stuck in a colorless and stale world.

These are the stories that can guide us and inspire us and give us the faith and motivation we need. Throughout time, there is an amazing legacy of radical belief and radical behavior. Endless stories have already been written.

A radical belief system may require you to be willing to remain committed to your convictions and stay steadfast in your goals no matter what "facts" appear to stand in your way.

Imagine a world full of people who wake up every day and look forward to leaving a mark.

We have always thought of our father as a man with a radical belief system. More importantly, we knew he was fiercely committed to his beliefs. There was no giving up and no wavering when this man decided to go all-in. We remember when he saw an opportunity to save the lives of countless people with serious injuries or ailments who had to be transported from outlying areas that lacked high-quality hospitals to receive better medical care. However, the length of the journey was actually killing them. He knew how to make a difference and was compelled to improve treatment protocol and transportation in hospitals across the world, even if it maxed out every one of his credit cards.

As a physician at the University of Virginia Hospital in the early 1980s, our father first noticed there was no adequate care offered to those with serious burns. So he drove the university to fix the situation and founded the Burn Unit. But even then his job was not done. He realized that the transport of these seriously burned patients also put them at risk and often led to their death. The most serious cases would be transported by ambulance to the UVA healthcare system. However, because of the fragility of these patients, the extensive travel time would put them at enormous risk for infections and complications. The only solution was to find a quicker way to transport patients.

While it may be the standard today in the medical industry, there was a time when helicopters or medi-planes were simply not accessible for emergency healthcare. But our dad knew they could save his patients' lives. So he pushed for funding to have helicopters available to transport the patients that were most in need. Initially, and for years to come, the healthcare system refused his requests. But one day enough was enough.

Dad heard about a burn victim who was eight hours away by ambulance from the UVA hospital. He knew the patient would never make it. So he took it upon himself to make the difference. He took out his credit card and rented a plane to transport the patient and ultimately saved his life. He put that receipt from his personal credit card in an expense report and gave it to the University of Virginia. The head of the hospital said,

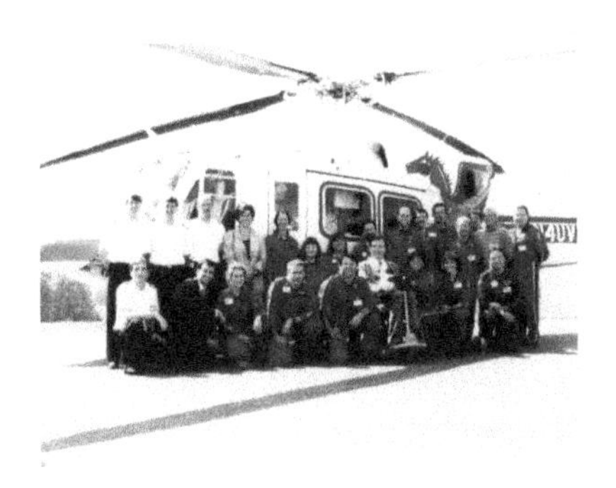

Our Dad in action in the field

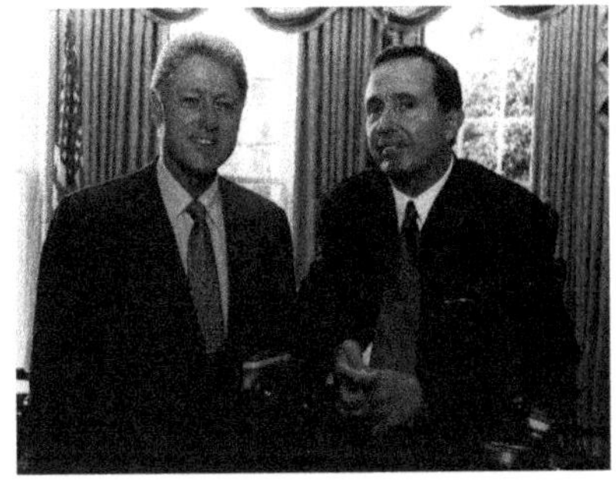

Bill Clinton with Our Dad

"Dr. Edlich, are you planning on doing this again?" Dad said, "You betcha." He was going to continue doing that until someone recognized the value in saving people's lives.

RADICAL *thought*

Radical belief anchors your vision of what's possible to be able to take radical action and make a radical difference.

Eventually, helicopter transportation became common practice for hospitals. This small but alarmingly expensive and radical practice of our father's turned into UVA Pegasus, a hospital-based air and ground transport service providing care to critically ill or injured patients. He stood when others stayed seated. And he crafted a belief system that served everyone involved.

Our father made a big impact in the medical world. He left a dent, one that made a large change and left a lasting and impactful impression. Radical belief simply calls you to see what is not yet visible to give you the drive to act on your conviction.

RADICAL *thought*

A whisper turns into a conversation, which turns into a belief that then manifests into committed conviction, which then becomes a reality.

Being a difference at any level makes a difference at all levels. So start by looking to where you can leave a dent. And then believe. Believe like you've never believed before. And use that radical belief to propel and accelerate you in the direction of your purpose, always remembering that nothing will open more doors and blast through more obstacles than committed conviction.

BUILDING BELIEF

We don't all have the foundations and immediate strengths to create and implement a radical belief system. But rest assured there are ways to improve the one you have.

We always tell people that to build a more radical belief system you have to take three critical but straightforward steps:

1. *Identify the landscape of your belief – know what you believe today*

2. *Craft beliefs that will serve you – adopt empowering beliefs*

3. *Surround yourself with people who support your beliefs*

We have a conscious and subconscious mind. We are constantly filtering and attracting new information into our lives, and our beliefs (which live in our subconscious) represent the most powerful partner or enemy in the reality we see in our life today. Therefore, we must identify and examine the beliefs that live in our subconscious, write them down, and then determine if a certain belief does or does not support what we want.

If a belief does not support and reflect the vision of what we want, we need to rewrite, change, and adopt a belief that does serve our desired outcome.

After replacing the faulty and disempowering belief with one that supports us, we should use repetition as a tool to fortify this belief and be mindful not to slide back to that long-held belief that takes us away from that which we desire.

So with this in mind, the next section will help you to become the master of your beliefs and paradigms. We break it down into bite size pieces for you to easily digest and create lasting results.

IDENTIFY THE LANDSCAPE OF YOUR BELIEF

This is the first step in mastering your beliefs.

As we discussed, many times we aren't even aware of where our belief systems fall. Left or right, up or down, vertical or horizontal. We all have a different set of beliefs that often dictate the manner in which we view the world. Many of these beliefs were embedded in our minds during childhood. Clearly, our parents' views and beliefs played a substantial role in how we see the world. But as we separate from our childhood and mature, our beliefs develop, change, and grow. What was once acceptable may not be any longer. What was once our norm may have considerably changed or not. Time allows for development, and it certainly promotes growth.

One of the greatest secrets to success is having clarity around your beliefs. Frankly, you either know what you believe in or you don't. Belief is cut and dry. There should never be any gray. If you want to build a belief system that supports your goals, you have to uncover what your beliefs are.

A Radical To-Do: Put a pen to paper and write down exactly what you believe. You may be surprised at what beliefs you own that do not offer the space to create what you want. When you take the time to examine your beliefs, you may be surprised at what you find.

What are your beliefs? Go ahead, you have come this far. Write them down: the good, the bad, and the ugly. Then take a look and know that these are only the ones you could come up with on command. These are the easy ones. They are the tip of your belief iceberg that makes itself known. There are far deeper, less prominent ones that drive you unconsciously and may be taking you down a road that you do not want to travel.

When these disempowering beliefs crop up, ask yourself the following question:

Is that really true?

Challenge your negative beliefs and aggressively embrace evidence that supports new ones that take you down the road to what you desire.

Set aside a moment and write the following statements:

I believe that:

Love is…

Money is…

I am…

Work is…

Life is…

Luck is…

Friends are…

Weight is…

Beauty is…

My body is…

Age is…

My career is…

My friends are…

My health is…

Time is…

I believe in…

Jot down the first things that come into your mind. That is your gut or your intuition at work. It will allow those clearly defined beliefs to surface. Next, begin to dive deeper. Consider your family, friends, profession, hobbies, religion, and any other core values. Take the time to analyze at a more profound level that which you hold dear. With that list in front of you, debate it. Discuss the pros and cons of each belief or value, and do your best to make an argument as to why they should stay or go. This process of evaluation will help you to separate the weak from the strong and ultimately cement your belief system. Living your life without a clearly defined belief system is tantamount to sailing without a map, or hiking an unknown mountain without a compass. Radical belief calls for basic planning. Exposing a belief system is as important as fighting against those who don't support you and your goals.

If you don't plan for what's to come, then you will ultimately get what life gives you.

CRAFT BELIEFS THAT SERVE YOU

The next step to building better beliefs is to *craft beliefs that will serve you.* Many times your beliefs are the antennae that attract your success. You will always find a way to support your beliefs as truth. So why wouldn't you choose beliefs that will attract things that support you and introduce the energy you need in your life to get where you want to go?

For example, let's assume you are a single woman, forty-five years of age, looking for the right partner. If you carried the belief that "women over forty don't have a chance because men want the younger women," you'll never be primed to find the right person. That limiting belief will always sabotage you and create hurdles along your journey.

If you keep up with the negative talk, it is difficult to build a strong belief system. We hear women say, "A divorcee with three kids is not very desirable; what man wants that baggage?" With that belief, you will never allow yourself the opportunity to take advantage of getting set-up, meeting new people, and dating. We know numerous men who crave family and children. The landscape of your belief system will create pinnacles you can never surmount. The reality is that you create your own landscape. You are the gardener and have ultimate control of your destiny. The world will mirror and reflect your beliefs.

RADICAL thought | Whatever you are seeing before you in your life is the result of your beliefs, good and bad.

There is an endless list of belief systems that do not support your radical life and actually sabotage you. They usually begin with words like: I can't, I won't, I am not. Often we give teeth to our beliefs. We find ways to make them truths, and they then become part of our fabric. If you change those beliefs, you'll begin to see numerous examples appear to prove their validity. If you believe you live in a world filled with caring and compassionate people, you will find those practices everywhere you look. But if you live in a dark world, always feeling like people are inherently selfish and cold-hearted, the world will act as your mirror, showing you a dismal reflection.

We are reminded of the studies conducted by scientists about conditioning and behavior. They had an open jar with no lid that they put flies in. As you might guess, the flies kept flying out. Then they put these same flies in a jar with an aerated lid on it for a day; the flies were trapped and could not get out. Then the following day the scientists used a screen on the top instead of a lid so the flies could feel the full effect of the air. The flies were still trapped. Finally, they removed the lids and left the top open to allow the flies the freedom to fly out.

Not only did they not fly out, they didn't even flutter their wings and try.

Why? The flies no longer believed that free flight was possible.

The same is true for us. Whatever we believe will prove true. So it is important to keep focused on beliefs that support us on our journey. We must know that the ceiling will be lifted when we make it so. No matter

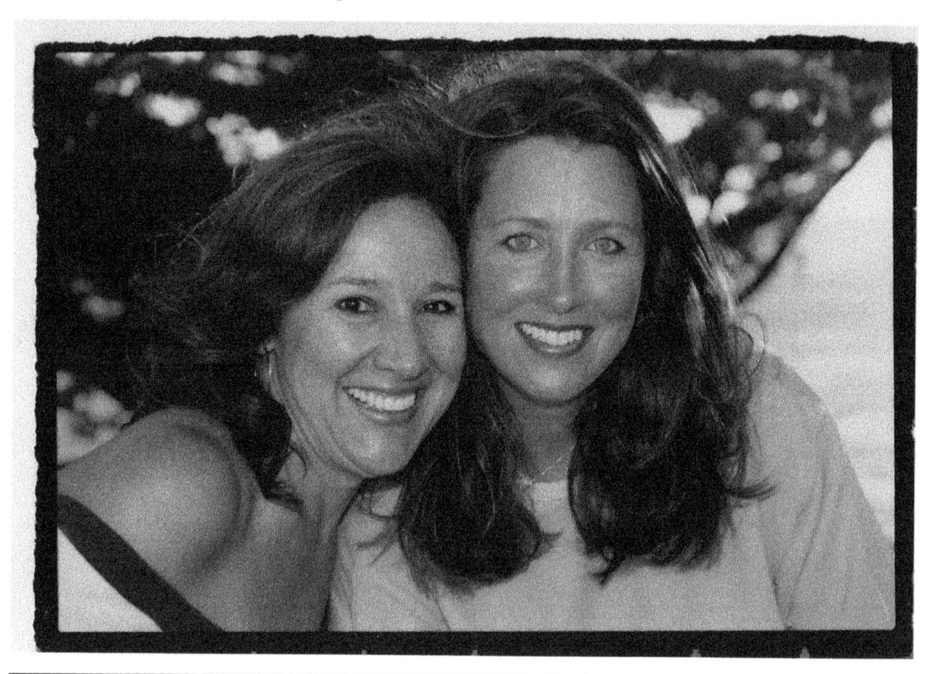

Liz and Maria (Liz age 32) (Maria age 47) in Malibu

how many experiences we have had where we failed, or how many people in our life have told us that it's not possible and that is just the way it is—know that these are limiting belief systems. Choose a different belief and keep going.

SURROUND YOURSELF WITH PEOPLE WHO SUPPORT YOUR POSITIVE BELIEFS

To build and support a life-changing belief system, we have to *surround ourselves with those who align with our beliefs and goals.* We call this creating your Radical Dream Team. While we touched on this in the previous chapter, it is important to expand on the notion that your belief system should be in complete alignment with those you welcome into your life. Sometimes you are strong enough to be the light, but other times you may need to borrow the belief other people have in you. When you don't entirely believe in the ability to succeed in your goals, take a moment to look around, lean on your support system, and absorb the faith others have in you, using it as a steppingstone to digest and adopt a powerful belief that serves you. Rely on that Radical Dream Team. It's often that small shove or nudge that helps to get you over the hump.

We need to bombard our conscious and subconscious with positive and affirming messages to outweigh the old beliefs that keep us stuck exactly where we are.

RADICAL *thought*

Sharon Lowe, "Nothing will stop the person with the right attitude, nothing will help the person with the wrong one."

We often hear the story of the woman in an abusive relationship. Her current boyfriend is a good-looking package and successful on the outside. But behind closed doors he is a drinker, cheater, and gambler who treats her with sporadic kindness, especially when he is trying to win her back – the infamous seduction/abandonment trap. High highs and low lows, with a promise for better days and a dreamier future.

One day she finally decides that enough is enough, breaks up with him, and works to move on with her life. She recognizes that there was an unhealthy addictive quality to the relationship, which makes it challenging to let go and to be attracted to a different dynamic. Her subconscious beliefs keep her stuck, and her very survival depends on reprograming these beliefs to attract her heart's desire.

Liz: That story was not just "some woman," that was me.

It took everything I had to make a radical change. At that point I had to borrow someone else's belief in me, as I had allowed mine to be beaten down. One day after yet another episode of emotional abuse and feeling dejected, my friend Maria looked at me and just started to cry. "I can't take it anymore," she said. "I can't stand the way he treats you and what it does to you. You deserve so much better." Seeing her despair and love toward me shocked me into the reality that enough was enough. Even though I did not feel the confidence or love for myself at the moment, I borrowed some of her love and belief in me. I swore that I would change my negative normal.

I decided to make a radical change. I left him. I moved three thousand miles away and started a new life. I promised that I would never find myself in that situation again. I began to make a list. This list encompassed everything I wanted in my future love. It took all the bad qualities of my ex to truly shine the light on what I did not want, as well as what I was determined to have.

I wrote down that list and would read and reread it and keep the vision and picture of what I wanted front and center.

After that list, I met men who were not the perfect fit, but I was willing to go on a date if they carried most of the qualities on my extensive list. I forced myself to surround myself with only kind and high-quality men. Even if I didn't see a future with a particular man, I was always willing to take the chance and get used to a new normal. I was radically committed to the belief that I deserved and would have it all, regardless of how the landscape looked at the present moment.

RADICAL *thought*

At times we all need a hand-up, not a handout. Borrow someone's belief in you when yours is shaky.

As I continued to date, I eventually found myself attracted to men with the qualities on my list. I literally created a new normal for myself. I was no longer attracted to the bad-boy mentality that caused so much trouble in the past. It was important to learn a different way of being, a different way of responding, and a different way of feeling so that I could create my new normal. While I may have felt uncomfortable in my new reality, sticking to my list and goals began to create a healthier and more positive life. And it all started with borrowing the beliefs from a member of my Radical Dream Team, Maria Price.

The list is endless when I look at the people in my life who have believed in me and helped to instill in me what I know in my heart is possible. Unfortunately, old paradigms that undermine you are always there bubbling right under the surface, looking for their opportunity to shine again and cause you to slip back into doing things that keep you stuck and not living to your full potential.

RADICAL thought | Albert Einstein said, "The definition of insanity is doing the same thing again and again and expecting a different result."

It is our job to love ourselves enough to keep reinforcing what we truly desire, studying to attain knowledge, and surrounding ourselves with others to keep us on our path.

One thing you can bet on with absolute certainty: with every passing year, when you look back, you will be far more saddened by the things you did not do than by the things you did do. Seize the opportunity to be the best that you can be and own beliefs that support you.

RADICAL thought | Name it, claim it, and have it. Whatever you desire is waiting for you.

Patience is a fundamental requirement to achieve anything of great value or meaning. It is a necessary evil to get where you want to go. When you incorporate patience, you receive a sense of peace. Tell yourself, "I'm right where I need to be today. This is a process. I need to be patient with the process to get where I'm going. The process isn't always pretty, but I'm going to get there."

Creating a better belief system is not difficult. It simply calls for you to focus your time and attention on minor adjustments that can make substantial differences. The three integral pieces mentioned above will help you grow and develop a rock-solid and hyper-focused belief system. You should feel proud of your belief system and always work to tweak it and elevate it. A radical belief system is one with great conviction – conviction in yourself and conviction in the world as it operates around you. If you don't believe, you won't achieve.

Radical Recap:

When you are trying to create a strong Radical Belief system, always remember that:

1. Believe like you've never believed before. And use that radical belief to propel and accelerate you in the direction of your purpose, always remembering that nothing will open more doors and blast through more obstacles than committed conviction.

2. If you believe something will work, it often can. However, if you believe it won't work, it never really had a chance in the first place. Don't ever stop believing.

3. Belief is not an individual sport. It takes a village. Surround yourself with like-minded people who believe in you and in your vision.

4. Replace old and outdated beliefs with new and fresh ones. We need to bombard our conscious and subconscious with positive and affirming messages to outweigh the old beliefs that keep us stuck exactly where we are.

5. Uncover disempowering beliefs by writing them down and then rewrite beliefs that serve you.

Chapter 13: RADICAL COURAGE

Fear.

That was the singular emotion we both felt when making the difficult decision to move from the East Coast and the comforts of our family, friends, relationships, and careers to this crazy city in California. We were born and bred as East Coast girls and really didn't know what to expect when moving across the country to Hollywood. The thought of uprooting our lives and moving made us both slightly nauseous. We didn't know a soul and were both in dead-end relationships that were not supporting our growth and development personally or professionally. We were about to make a move from small-town America to the big and exciting city of Los Angeles.

Anxiety.

When the fear subsided, anxiety took hold. No matter how many times we reminded ourselves that this was our decision and the right move to make, it was hard to mute the voices that reminded us of the enormous mystery and unanswered questions.

Back and forth, back and forth, analyzing and reviewing the decision. Hoping that following this new road would lead to a successful outcome.

This was big. This was life-altering. Sure, we could always pack up our belongings and return home. That was always an option. But to do that would admit failure. And more importantly, it would place us back at the center of the unappealing status quo.

It wasn't an easy decision to conclude that packing up our lives and moving thousands of miles away was the right move. There was a lot of internal doubt. How could there not be? To that point in our lives, moving across country was the biggest risk we've ever assumed.

- *What if we were making the wrong decision?*
- *What if we didn't fit in?*
- *What if our family and friends at home harbored anger and felt abandoned?*
- *What if we couldn't find our way and rebuild our lives and make a living?*

We knew the present situation had to change. It wasn't working and it wasn't supporting our lives. We made this radical decision at different times and at different ages in our lives. We both buckled our seatbelt for the adventure, drowning in a sea of unanswered questions.

Into the abyss.

Into the unknown.

Into La-La Land.

But we saw it through. We each loaded up our cars, turned the key, backed out of the driveway, and put the pedal to the metal, and with every passing mile and every passing day, left the comforts of the known and status quo behind. As we edged closer to Los Angeles, our fear began to transform into something else. It was slowly replaced with hope, with opportunity. We still had no clue what the journey had in store, but we rolled down our windows, took in the fresh air, and felt reinvigorated and ready to experience that which was yet to come.

Courageous.

Looking back, that was the word to describe our journey. Courage is an essential part of the prescription. There was no turning back. Good, bad, or indifferent, we had just made a radically courageous decision. At its most fundamental level, radical courage is really about overcoming fear; it is about looking around you, at your boundaries and comfort zone, and then completely disregarding them.

- *It is about getting in the car, turning on the engine, and driving in the direction of your dreams. It is about cracking the windows so the fresh air of opportunity can blow in. Every day welcomes in an exciting opportunity to get just a little uncomfortable.*

- *Radical courage is the courage to listen and take heed when you hear that inner voice.*
- *Radical courage is the courage to trust people you do not know.*
- *Radical courage is the courage to take a chance, not really knowing what may happen.*
- *Radical courage is the courage to believe in people, when life hasn't always rewarded that belief.*
- *Radical courage is the courage to believe that you can and will create the life you love.*
- *And radical courage is the courage to follow your dreams and your vision, even when doing so may be just a little uncomfortable.*

Radical courage is both a learned behavior *and* a conscious decision. We believe the courage to follow your intuition is one of the most important factors in having everything that you desire. The little clues that take you off your predictable route may lead you to your riches. Riches can be more than just money. They can be your relationships and friendships, or a job that you are passionate about. The list is endless. The riches are everywhere.

RADICAL *fact*

The word courage comes from "cor" in Latin, which means heart. It is a common metaphor for inner strength.[12]

The key is to listen to that little voice inside you so you can be open to it and allow it to take you down those magical roads. Then you just have to be courageous enough to take action on what the little voice tells you.

Radical courage is setting aside all the "what if's" and jumping in, knowing that you will somehow see it through. To propel us to take courageous steps we need to believe that where we are going is possible. That possibility will be the fuel to drive us into action.

Sometimes our engines need a different type of fuel. Not the fuel that was in our cars when we left for California. Rather, the fuel that was in our souls that pushed us to leave. That type of fuel is intangible and not easy to quantify. But it is the fuel that separates people from one another. It is what fuels radical courage. When we left for California, fear was replaced with excitement—the excitement of a new opportunity and the fuel to create a new *us*, a new life.

Courage can be quiet or quite loud.

Courage can be internal or external.

Courage can be subtle or in your face.

Courage can be personal or professional.

Courage can make a difference to just one person or many people.

Courage can be learned and even taught.

COURAGE IS OVERCOMING FEAR

When we think of courage, we think of overcoming fear. In life, and to be radically courageous, you have to believe in yourself enough to take risks. That belief often comes from clarity and vision. It is far easier to believe that something is possible when you can close your eyes and see it come to life. That imagination is what can help you along in your journey.

Once focus and imagination replace fear, you will reach the level of clarity needed to courageously put one foot in front of the other.

Rachel: When I reflect on my life, I never thought I would be going through a divorce for a second time. Hard to admit, and it weighs heavy on my heart. Do I want to write and share this part of my life in this book? Not particularly. Then why? Because I know I'm not alone and that my journey could help someone else who may be challenged with some of the same conversations I had in my head, self-doubt, fear, anxiety, worry, loss, pain, panic, sadness, and an overwhelming fear of failing.

As I was walking up to the edge of making the decision to divorce, negative and defeating talk tracks beckoned me to back away. *What are you thinking? Why would you do this? The kids? The money? The change? What if you are alone? What if you are wrong? Shouldn't you try again? Is this really a good time?* I could find a million good reasons not to divorce rather than jump into a pool of uncharted water.

RADICAL *fact*

Approximately 40 percent of fears and worries never materialize, 30 percent of your fears are about your past, and about 22 percent are about things that are not important in the big picture.

We have plenty of negative chatting in our mind to tell us why we cannot make it and why we will fail on our journey. And we may hate every step as we walk up to that decision and finally jump in the water and scream, "Okay, I said it, I did it, I am on my way... but how? I have never swum in this lane before."

I don't want to take you through all the details. Let's just say that I believe fully in marriage and being in a committed relationship. Family is the *most* important thing to me so dismantling mine was the hardest thing I have ever done. Especially my most recent divorce. No one wins in divorce, and we all go into marriage believing that it is forever. I thought I had gotten it right, which I did for several years. We have known each other for twenty years and were best friends, soul mates, and shared a very deep connected love, which made my decision to leave one that took me several years to do. It didn't happen overnight, but after years of questioning the impact it would have on the children, my family, my future, and his future. Also it was hard to accept that I would have to start all over again.

The most heart-wrenching part was that it was an addiction that took him out of our family. He went through five back surgeries, and after the last surgery became dependent on prescription medication, which took his soul and the man I loved so much. Without the medication he was in pain, and with the medication he was high and out of pain but also out of touch with everyone around him. He felt alive and energetic with the children, but he wasn't the same amazing father with the filter of pain medication. A different, disconnected person would show up that took over the man I so loved. I'm a fighter, and I will fight to keep my family together almost to a fault.

Feeling guilt and shame daily about my children being separated, I delayed the inevitable. I would imagine my daughter crying and begging for us to be together and my son detaching and being upset with me for doing this twice to him. So I stayed and I stayed and I prayed for direction. My indecision was a decision, and I understood that. I couldn't complain about my situation because it was a choice. A choice I was making until I was willing to do something different. Until finally the pain of staying was too unbearable and I was empty inside. I just couldn't watch or have my children watch him fall apart again. On the brink of a nervous breakdown myself, I had to get courageous and know that this wasn't the life I wanted to live, nor was it what I wanted for my children. I needed to stand up for a healthy, safe, stress-free environment for all of us.

I had to visualize and have faith that the life I wanted was filled with laughter, partnership, support, hard work, balance, respect, love, family, friends, and connection. We all deserve that in our life. When I looked at my marriage I always looked at it like a pie: 80 percent great and 20 percent things to work on. The greatness always outweighed the negative. I considered myself lucky. Most people looked at our relationship wishing they had what we had. When it flip-flopped and became 90 percent hard and 10 percent okay for several years, I knew I needed to respect myself more than to subject myself or my kids to this pie. I believed that when we split we still had a chance, though I knew I wasn't going to go backwards and replay the same situation; something major would have to change for the both of us. I focused on my goal of creating a stress-free environment and had to take baby steps to get there. When doubt came over me, I focused on creating peace around me, focused on caring for my kids, and recognized that I couldn't have that with him at this point. So I filed for divorce.

Today my children are doing great, well adjusted but never perfect. I continue to visualize happiness and health for their dad and believe that he will find his way back to create a life he loves. It will take a great deal of courage and commitment for him to get himself there.

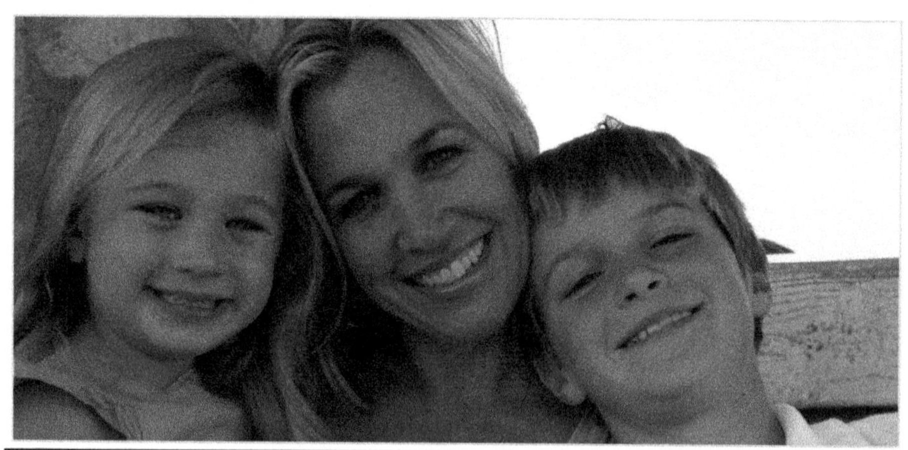

Rachel Edlich with her kids Sophia and Forrest

Courage. It's not easy to stay the course and take those steps toward a better you and a better life. It takes a lot of faith and can only happen one day at a time, one step at a time, one minute at a time. It takes believing and being committed to a vision that supports you and being willing to abandon that which does not.

KNOCK DOWN YOUR TERROR BARRIERS

Bob Proctor always says, "The radical individual is courageous." They go where they want to go even though they've never been there. Fear doesn't stop them. You see, radical individuals have fear; they just don't let it stop them. They go where most people have never been. And that's what makes them radical.

When we go ahead, the courage and the ability to focus enables us to knock down what Bob calls the terror barriers. The average individual lets the terror barriers stop them, and they go back into bondage and that's where they stay. They sort of tiptoe through life hoping they make it safely to death. They never step out and bet on the surest thing in the world, which is themselves. They don't need other people to guide them. That doesn't mean they don't look for guidance – they do. They look for help.

The radical person is a super-serious student. They're always studying something they don't understand, because they want to gain understanding. They realize understanding only comes one way – through study. They realize that understanding is the polar opposite to doubt and worry. So when doubt and worry strike, they know it's because there's something they don't understand and they get studying. They eliminate the doubt and the worry, which lead to fear, and they go on to understanding, which leads to faith and expression.

The radical individual goes where they've never been before. They don't let the darkness of the future stop them. They have the courage to move forward into the unknown and unpredictable.

Steve Jobs said that "you cannot connect the dots looking forward, you can only connect them looking backwards." So you have to trust that the dots will somehow connect in the future and keep moving forward.

Courage is the ability to capture and then maintain the vision of your goals and desired life, even when you feel a little uneasy in the process. When we left for California, fear was replaced with excitement – the excitement of a new opportunity. Even the act of leaving a marriage can be seen through the lens of fear, or the lens of a vision of what is possible…the dream you hold clear and dear in your mind's eye.

We often relate courage to the act of overcoming the fear of something: fear of the unknown, fear of the known, or just the fear of something that tripped us up in the past. Maybe it is the fear that comes from a bad experience, or failure, or the scars from getting burned by life. That fear is a limiter. It prevents us from moving forward in our respective lives and puts a low ceiling on our ability to succeed. Just like courage, fear also comes in many different shapes and sizes.

TAKING RISKS + LEARNING FROM MISTAKES = CREATING YOUR DREAMS

Risk taking is one of the key factors in achieving success. Making mistakes is part of the process, and those who can be agile and keep going and risk again win and create their dreams.

Our dear friend Samantha Hart, one of our senior brand advisors, shares a similar view of risk taking. In addition to being a brand visionary for Radical Skincare, Samantha is founder of Foundation Content, an award-winning, full-service production company. She has won numerous awards for both her creative writing and design including the prestigious Gold Hugo award for her work on United Way. We are blessed to have such a radical, courageous woman on our team.

Before starting Foundation Content, Samantha had a successful career in the entertainment industry, which began under the mentorship of David Geffen working on projects for bands such as Nirvana, Guns 'N Roses, and Aerosmith. She went on to become creative director at Gramercy Pictures (now Focus Films).

Samantha's creative vision brought prominence to such independent features as *Dead Man Walking, Fargo, The Usual Suspects,* and *Four*

Weddings and a Funeral. She continued her successful run of hits at Fox Searchlight with *Waking Ned Devine* and *Boys Don't Cry* before moving to Universal Pictures as senior vice president of marketing and advertising.

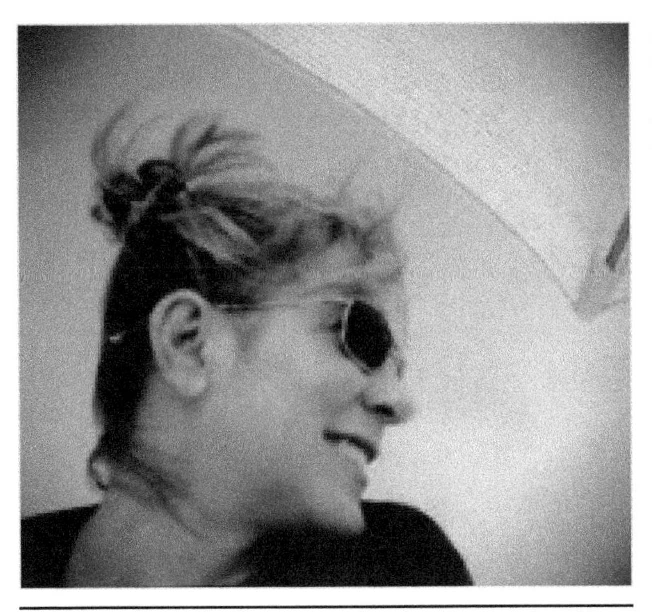

Producer, Creative director and writer Samantha Hart

Samantha believes that "achieving a radical life means being authentic, taking chances, and taking risks in yourself. Don't be afraid to say what you want to do and then pursue it. Don't be afraid to go in another direction if it's not working for you. Many people I've met log onto the idea of 'I want to do this.' But when 'this' doesn't happen for them, they then feel like a failure. Instead, we should think 'Well, I pursued this, it wasn't for me, but along the way I learned an important lesson. Failure isn't about falling down it is about staying down. As long as you have learned something from your experiences it is far from failure.'"

RADICAL *thought*

FEAR: **F**alse **E**vidence **A**ppearing **R**eal.

She continues: "Great things happen when you believe that the outcome is always going to have a deeper meaning or resonate on another level in your life. If you choose to live life positively, then things can happen for a reason. When things don't go as planned, you know you had to have this experience to get to the positive part. Courage is taking the risk knowing there's a chance of missing the mark because even if you miss, things will always work out for the best. We must take the radical leap and take chances – both externally and internally."

Muhammad Ali said, "He who is not courageous enough to take risks will accomplish nothing in life." So maybe courage is anything that involves removing yourself from the warmth and coziness of your everyday life and getting just a little uncomfortable.

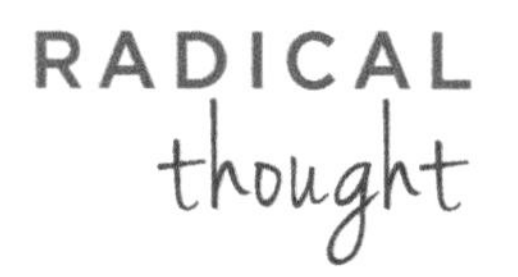

Courage is tapping into and anchoring your life in a belief system that says anything is possible. T.S. Eliot said, "Only those who will risk going too far can possibly find out how far one can go."

So it begs the question:

- *How far will you go?*
- *What is it that you want more than the fear of what is holding you back?*
- *What things would you do differently if you didn't fear doing them?*
- *What does it cost you not to do these things that you want?*
- *When you look back at your life, will you regret letting your fear win over your wants?*
- *What will you gain by getting over the fear and doing what you really want?*
- *When you look back at your life and think of things you were afraid of happening, how many actually happened?*
- *How many of these predictions were False Evidence Appearing Real?*

LIFE WITH THE BIRDS

One of our favorite people, Tippi Hedren, has shown us just how powerful pushing yourself out of your comfort zone can be. Against all odds, the beautiful twenty-year-old who bought a ticket to New York City in 1950, with lofty dreams of being a model, actually became one! She spent a decade reigning at the premier Ford Agency as one of their most coveted models – even appearing on the cover of *Life* magazine. She had everything she dreamed of in the palm of her hand: success, a husband, and a beautiful daughter.

Until it was snatched away . . .

Suddenly she was divorced, her modeling career was over, and she was a single mom starting over in Los Angeles with four-year-old Melanie in tow. Tippi knew she had to recreate her life, but her options were extremely limited. Her answer came on Friday the 13th, October 1961, in the form of a mysterious phone call from an executive at Universal Studios. "Are you the girl from those Sego diet drink commercials? A well-known director/producer is interested in you."

Become an actress?

Could she do it?

The next call resulted in a meeting with Lew Wasserman at MCA. The legendary theatrical agent who represented everyone from Ronald Reagan to Jimmy Stewart to Bette Davis told her, "Alfred Hitchcock wants to sign you to a contract."

Tippi stared at him with disbelief. "*Alfred Hitchcock* wants me to appear in a movie?"

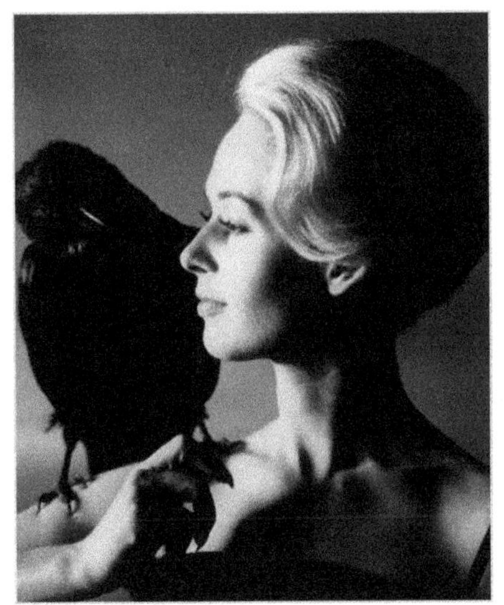

Actress Tippi Hedren in The Birds

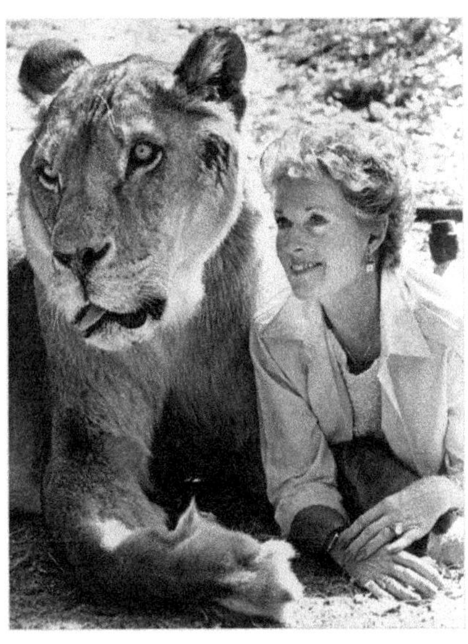

Actress Tippi Hedren with her lion friend as part of her Shambala Foundation: Shambala.org

Lew nodded. "Alfred watches the *Today Show* every morning. The girl in the Sego diet drink commercials has fascinated him. When he saw you in those commercials he decided you would be better served as a star in his films. He is quite fascinated with you. If you agree to the terms, we'll go over the details."

Tippi drew on the same courage that had put her on a plane at age twenty as she reached for the papers to sign them. She was introduced to Alfred Hitchcock the same day – entering what she believed was a magical time of her life.

"About three weeks after the test I was invited to Chasen's, an incredibly chic restaurant. When I sat down he laid a wrapped package in front of me from Gump's, a beautiful gift shop in San Francisco. I opened it to discover a beautiful gold-and-pearl brooch of three birds in flight. I looked up in awe as Hitchcock told me I was to play Melanie Daniels in *The Birds*. I did what any woman would do; I started to cry. Mrs. Hitchcock was crying, and even Lew Wasserman, the tough-as-nails agent, had a tear rolling down his cheek. Alfred sat there looking quite pleased with himself."

Tippi had gone from being a desperate single mother at the tail end of a modeling career to Hitchcock's leading lady. What could be more perfect? Tippi, determined to justify Hitchcock's faith in her, did whatever he asked. During the filming of *The Birds,* she often went face-to-face with the feathered creatures, brushing off her injuries as "scratches and that sort of thing." She had been given the chance of a lifetime; she would do nothing to jeopardize it.

The last scene of the infamous film almost pushed her beyond the bounds of her courage. She had been told mechanical birds would be flung at her. Instead, five live seagulls were harnessed to different parts of her body, while dozens of shrieking birds were flung at her. Finally, when the bird tied onto her shoulder gouged her cheek with its beak, narrowly missing her eye, she reached her limit.

"Please remove the birds," she said, somehow maintaining her calm. "I think I've had enough of this." Tippi has no memory of the drive home, the weekend that followed, or driving herself to the set on Monday morning. When she arrived at the studio, she passed out on her chaise lounge and could not be woken. Her doctors diagnosed her with exhaustion and prescribed a week off from the film.

Hitchcock refused. Somehow Tippi finished the film in a state of torment that only added to the quality of the performance.

Despite Hitchcock's torturous expectations, Tippi was thrilled to be asked to play the title character in Hitchcock's next film, *Marnie.* Unfortunately, while she was experiencing heady success as an actress, the torment of her behind-the-scenes life with Hitchcock was becoming unbearable. His fascination with Tippi had morphed into an obsession that demanded he control every aspect of her life – what she wore, what she ate, what she drank. She was uncomfortably aware that he was watching her all the time. She dreamed of walking away but was desperately afraid she would be blacklisted and unable to find work.

The unbearable became impossible when Hitchcock called her into a meeting, looked at her, and said calmly, "From this time on, I expect you to make yourself sexually available and accessible to me – however, whenever, and wherever I want."

Tippi's great courage rose again, drowning out all fear. "I will never do those things," she said firmly. "I want out of my contract. We are done."

Hitchcock refused, promising to destroy her career for her stand. Her inexperience had made her sign a contract that basically gave the director control of her life and her future. For two years he paid her weekly to do nothing, while he also turned down every film offer that came her way. Tippi had enough money to support Melanie, but for all intents and purposes her acting career was finished.

Two years would pass before Hitchcock finally sold her contract to Universal Studios, which two years later released her from contract – giving her back control of her decisions and her future. Her refusal to compromise herself also led her in an entirely new direction.

In 1972, Tippi Hedren founded an animal rescue organization, Roar Foundation and Shambala Preserve, located outside Los Angeles.[13] Shortly thereafter, she reinvented herself and embraced her passion for exotic cats and animals. She saved them and they saved her.

Courage is walking away when it may not be the popular decision. And for Tippi, the courage to close one door, which opened another, has brought immeasurable joy in giving back to these beautiful creatures in need. She found herself unbelievably fulfilled and reconnected with her happiness, which she lost during her time in film.

Remember what we said earlier?

Whether this prison is of your own making or someone else's, the only way to escape is to make the difficult decision to leave something or someone important to you behind.

Tippi Hedren embodies this truth. She courageously walked away from abuse and humiliation. Her step of courage did nothing but strengthen her courage to do as much with her life as possible as she continued moving forward. Moviegoers and TV watchers thank her, but the most important thanks come from the animals she has rescued.

Aristotle said, "You will never do anything in this world without courage." In life, we all want guarantees. But life really offers few of them. As for us, we subscribe to the idea that facing fears and overcoming them is courageous. It doesn't matter how big or small the fear (or the implications) may be. Big or small, overcoming any type of fear is radically courageous. Tippi had it all. But it was the courage she exhibited in stepping away from a life of financial security and fame that may be her greatest legacy.

S-V-P: STRENGTH, VISION, AND PERSEVERANCE

For us, courage has three pillars: strength, vision, and perseverance. As seen above, it truly does come in many different shapes and sizes. When these three qualities intersect, amazing things occur.

Strength. We are all born with strength. It is life's obstacles and adversity that often break us down and weaken our undeniable strength.

Rather than allowing your struggles to break you down, begin the journey of turning these negatives into positives. As you overcome adversity, allow the experience to build you up and strengthen your dedication and determination. Strength can be found everywhere. It can be seen in children's hospitals where small hearts and souls fight terrible illnesses just to stay live; it is present in the people who lose their loved ones to acts of violence; it is apparent in those people who rebuild their lives and communities after natural disaster hits; it is found in the women and children who leave abusive relationships; and of course strength can be found in each of us as we navigate life and handle the trials we face with amazing grace and a positive attitude. Strength is in you, now own it.

Vision. Vision is the ability to see the end result before it occurs. Visionaries are those people who can see through the small pinhole or the dimly lit hallway. They often see where others cannot. Vision isn't always easy and requires a willingness to focus on that which has yet to be seen. Oftentimes, vision is that which allows courage to rise within us. When you have a steadfast belief that your vision will eventually become your reality, it will help you to secure the courage to make the move you need to make.

Helen Keller said, "The only thing worse than being blind is having sight but no vision."

Most of us have the ability to see what is in front of us. But the trick is to visualize what we want in the future. You will be courageous when you capture a glimpse of that picture and own that as the reality you are committed to creating.

Why?

Because once you believe that what you envision will eventually manifest itself in your life, the courage to move forward will arrive.

Perseverance. Once you have harnessed your strength and vision of what's possible, you must have the perseverance to do whatever it takes to reach your goal. Be resilient, and have that never give-up attitude, the kind of swagger that allows you to bounce back from adversity when it hits you right in the mouth. Julie Andrews reminds us, "Perseverance is failing nineteen times and succeeding the twentieth."

We'd agree that falling down is simply part of the game. But how many times you get up is what separates those who succeed from those who fail. It's a willingness to dust yourself off and get back up to forge ahead. It is a must. Because you never know how close you are to the finish line until you get there.

Courage requires an enormous amount of perseverance. And oftentimes the most courageous people around us are those who are simply willing to persevere. So when you think of perseverance, think of that undeniable desire to continue putting one foot in front of the other in the face of relentless force pushing you in the opposite direction.

Danette Eilenberg, Radical sister on a mission, says, "If you feel like you are neck deep in doo-doo, don't worry, soon it will become fertilizer to grow your dreams!" We love that quote because it is just the way life is. We just need to see the challenges as fertilizer to live and grow by.

Radical courage is found at the intersection of strength, vision, and perseverance. It is not always easy to be strong, to maintain vision, and to persevere when your journey takes a turn for the worse. But we assure you that if you can harness just one of these qualities, the other two will follow and accompany you on your voyage to creating the life you love.

RADICAL COURAGE IN ACTION

We all need an action plan to build, increase, and maintain our radical courage. For us, we have taken three steps to help construct a high level of courage and overcome the fear that can stop us from moving forward. And if we rely on these three fundamental principles throughout our lives, we find that we are constantly working and moving toward a fulfilling life with radical courage.

Step 1 – Empower Yourself. You can be your worst enemy or your finest advocate. Building radical courage calls for you to empower yourself, from the start of your day. Think about those first few minutes of your day, the ones where you are lying in bed, contemplating whether you should jump out of bed and prepare for the day, or lie there, letting the minutes pass you by. We all know people who start their days defeated, unable to hit the ground running. They stall out before they even begin rolling. It happened to us. We would talk ourselves out of anything and everything, but especially starting the day.

But now we work to courageously start our day. When the alarm goes off, we jump out of the bed like a rocket. No time to think. No time to evaluate or analyze. Just a simple yet determined movement. This simple act eliminates the time to negotiate with that inner voice and justify inaction.

With empowerment comes happiness, but as Melanie Griffith shares, you must have the courage to put yourself first. She says, "You've got to fight or true happiness. Nobody can give it to you. You can't look to someone else for your happiness. Happiness absolutely has to come from within. I think the radical choice that has been the hardest choice of my life was to actually put myself first. To be feminine; I am not a feminist, but I am feminine. I'm a woman and I'm powerful." Express your magnificence and share it with the world.

Step 2 – Chunk It Down. The second step to inviting radical courage into your life is to realize that radical courage isn't a straight line, but more like a ladder. It occurs in small steps, and one step at a time. Far too many people believe it has to happen overnight. They think it has to be big steps. The truth is that nothing radical ever happened as a flash of lightning. So consider chunking your courage down into easy and manageable steps. When you are considering something as life changing as moving to a new city, or leaving a marriage or a job, feeling overwhelmed is certainly normal.

The truth is that nothing great was ever accomplished without a series of small victories. It takes enormous courage to make such a drastic life-change. But if you chunk it down and take one step at a time, you'll find more clarity and instill a sharper vision and greater belief system. A radical belief system fueled by courage will support the notion that you can and will succeed. When you take the time to chunk it down and plan the bites, you'll eventually find that you have created a much more manageable and palatable situation. You can change your life and you can even change the world. Let what you want be bigger than your fear of doing it.

Step 3 – Avoid Courage-Killers. The final step to creating and manifesting radical courage is to avoid the courage-killers. Unfortunately, they are everywhere.

RADICAL thought

Courage is like a candle. It needs oxygen to burn bright. When you take away its oxygen, it will begin to flicker and eventually burn out. Courage-killers are those things that suck the oxygen out of the air and eventually extinguish your inner desire.

One example of a courage-killer is resignation; the feeling of hopeless resignation, of being resigned to the notion that nothing is possible and the status quo will always remain. Courage-killers are often limiting beliefs.

You have to reach for something bigger than yourself with purpose and passion. Your dreams should always be designed to fulfill your heart and soul while exciting you. It is that excitement that will give you the energy to keep going no matter what. Far too often, people set goals without meaning. And when they reach them, they wonder why they wanted it in the first place. That is not you. You are bigger than that.

Martin Luther King Jr. said, "Faith is taking the first step even though you don't see the whole staircase."

Radical courage is centered on any opportunity to overcome fear and get yourself out of your comfort zone to achieve your dream. Small steps lead to big results. Make a list of those things in your life that cause discomfort or fear. And then take them one at a time, and start to move in the direction of believing you can. Compartmentalize your fears, put them in a box, get about your business, and move past them.

Fear does not serve you when it gets in the way of pursuing your dream or, at the most basic level, pursuing being in a better space or place. It doesn't have to be an act as large as moving across the country. It is the small victories that matter. And you have the ability to win these small battles every day you embrace your life. Ask yourself the question: If I had to do it all again, what would I do differently? Know that today is a new day and tomorrow is an opportunity to embrace your life and have no excuses or regrets. With that said, be radically fearless and know that:

Radical courage is yours for the taking.

Own it. Be it.

Because you can.

Radical Recap:

To help elevate your Radical Courage, always remember that:

1. Often times, fear precedes courage. It is like the smoke before a blazing hot fire. With that said, understand that where there is fear, there is an opportunity to succeed.

2. The radical individual goes where they've never been before. They don't let the darkness of the future stop them. They have the courage to move forward into the unknown and unpredictable.

3. Sometimes courage is walking away when it may not be the popular decision. The most courageous people know when they should stand up and when they should sit down.

4. Courage is putting one foot in front of the other because you can with no guarantees. Only focus on the opportunities to have a breakthrough and create your dream.

5. Courage requires faith. Surround yourself with those that bolster and support the belief of what is possible for your life.

Chapter 14:
RADICAL BEAUTY: INSIDE AND OUT

Being in the skincare industry, you would think that a chapter on beauty would be second nature and the easiest chapter in the book. But as we sat and looked at each other, with the task of sharing what beauty meant to us, we didn't know whether to laugh or cry. We knew it was an important part of the prescription, but we still felt challenged by its overall role. Beauty. Not easily definable by normal standards. For us, it truly required a different definition that stretched the mind by radical standards.

After interviewing hundreds of people in the last two years, we realized beauty was not simply based on looks, dress, or makeup. It had to do with what emanated from each person, act, or moment that left a lasting and beautiful impact on the world.

So one recent story that played in the forefront of our minds was a beautiful act from one sister to another. This act was partially known, partially unknown. It created environmental beauty, community beauty, and beautiful memories, and it spoke of love and giving, arriving unexpectedly and truly to the surprise of all. Radical beauty is the act of going above and beyond because you can and are willing to. It makes a difference and is beautiful. Since I (Liz) was on the giving end, I will share it from my perspective.

Liz: Over the past two or three years, Rachel has wanted to redecorate her home, purchase a couch that the kids could snuggle on in the family room together, create a less cluttered environment, update some furniture and fixtures, and organize the years stored away in the drawers so as to put them in their little boxes and create room for the new and beautiful, might we say. But as we all know, sometimes life just gets in the way.

Such a transformation becomes part of another to-do list, and then when you stack the priorities of family, work, school, sports, and plenty of other activities, there is very little room for a home remodel or redecoration. And so the days turned into weeks, weeks turned into months, and months turned into years; it never got done. So eventually I saw an opportunity and decided to do something about it.

I thought about my life, the money I have earned, the difference I wanted to make, and started thinking about what difference I could make in the lives of the people I love the most. What joy could I give to them, and then witness it firsthand? These are some of the questions to ask on a daily basis…

If not now, then when?

If not me, then who?

The answer that day was "it's up to me to act now."

It was Thanksgiving week and Rachel was taking the kids to the East Coast for their traditional holiday with cousins and family. I decided everything in life starts with a decision and then the unwavering commitment, passion, and perseverance to follow through with it.

So… I decided to remodel her home, from top to bottom in the four days she would be gone. Paint, redo ceilings, new furniture, and a huge snuggle couch, bedding, curtains, carpet cleaning, landscaping, rugs, hanging art from storage, and the overwhelming task of organizing closets and cabinets . . . YUCK! But it had to be done. And I was just the sister to do it.

I called a contractor friend and said, "I want to surprise my sis in a week and redo her home." After explaining my goals, he said okay. Boy was he in for a surprise. When we arrived at the house the morning we were scheduled to begin, he looked at me and said, "Are you kidding? There is no way we will finish all that you want to do in a week. And it's Thanksgiving week."

I could see his point. But in life, people will always tell you all of the rational reasons *why* something is not possible. What I needed to do was get radical in my approach. I would not stop until the job was done, and I would involve anyone and everyone in the opportunity to be part of something that mattered and would make a difference to someone I loved. So I enlisted Rachel's nanny Sabina, her son Kevin, his brother, and friend, my gardener, and eventually a community of loving help and kindness. The next thing I knew, we had a small army! Many of us were painting for the first time right next to professionals that are hired regularly by the Four Seasons hotel. My car looked like a moving van piled to the roof with loads from local stores.

Suffice it to say, we did it! Acting radically created a beautiful transformation that met my sister and her kids after their vacation with joy, glee, and tears of disbelief.

While I was in San Francisco running a Radical event, I had Rachel's closest friends there to film her reaction. It was one of the most beautiful moments of my life, knowing that I could make a radical difference in her life and in the life of her kids. The joy and warmth I experienced was amazing. I know she felt the same. That was beauty. That was rich. That was fulfilling. That created a glow and twinkle in my eyes and in hers. That is the beauty of being able to say a *Radical Yes* to the opportunity to create and experience beauty because you can.

Even better is that everyone involved felt a sense of community and accomplishment by being a part of something that really mattered. What started as a gift that I wanted to give to my sister touched many and turned into an inspiration that motivated them to join in and accomplish something remarkable and beautiful.

Everyone was lit up. They saw the difference, the excitement became pervasive, and everyone won.

So, the point of this story is that you'd think that two girls who started a skincare line would tell you that beauty is technical and skin-deep. For many, it may be. For us, beauty is something you feel. It is something you give to others. Radical beauty is inside out, rather than the alternative.

When we think of beauty, it is the long walks on a beach with a loved one; the sounds of your children playing and laughing together; the moments you share with your friends and family around a dinner table or in your living room; the unexpected surprise you can give your sister when she is out of town. Beauty is those sensitive yet fragile moments when connection occurs. Beauty surrounds us and every day offers an opportunity to project and introduce more beauty into the world.

BEAUTI-FEEL

Beauty is something you give to others. What makes you beautiful is how you care for and treat those around you. Beautiful people look to spread happiness and build people up. That is truly what beautiful people do. Beautiful people look for, in fact search for, the occasion to make others feel beautiful. To uplift them, love them, and make them more comfortable in their own skin.

Plenty of people assume that we have a traditional perception of beauty. We chalk it up to the fact that we have dedicated much of our adult years to creating products that help to make people appear more beautiful and solve skincare and confidence concerns. But the truth is that Radical Skincare was born from the heart. It came from the soul. It was built with the intention of improving the world by giving people what they wanted and then giving them what they needed to truly feel beautiful.

Therefore, our goal was never just to make people look beautiful; it was, much like our definition of beauty, to create a product line that makes women *feel* beautiful. Because how you feel is felt by the world. We wanted to give women and men a tool, a resource, to feel better about themselves. To transform and fade the blemishes or the wrinkles on their skin, so something much more powerful can rise to the top.

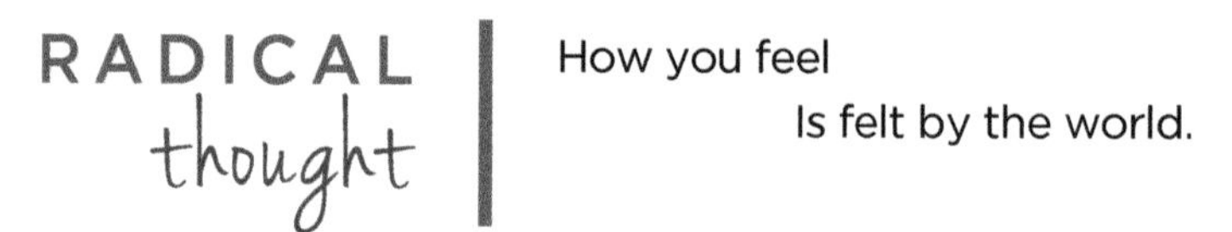

There is an absolute correlation between how you feel about yourself and how the world feels about you. When you radiate confidence, composure, and are ready to truly embrace life, you are able to give those exact same qualities to the people around you. You are better positioned to be a difference maker, a happiness provider, and a success builder when you *feel* good about yourself.

RADICAL *fact*

Studies have shown there are many benefits to self-confidence such as improved health, higher levels of satisfaction and happiness, increased performance, and positive social interactions.[14]

It is kind of silly, and sad at times, how we as women tie so much of our value to how we look. Our beauty has always been of utmost importance. For us, when we dealt with challenging skin conditions, we lost our confidence, our love of life, and our desire to get out there and smile. It wasn't proportionate to the problem, and there were far worse tragedies going on in the world. However, we couldn't help but let it impact who we were showing up as, or how we acted and felt.

What we learned is that many women had the same issues we did. In fact, at some point most women will allow how they look to affect how they feel. So if our Trylacel technology for skin improved how we felt and improved our ability to just get out there, why couldn't it play the same role for the rest of our gender? Our goal was not just to make women *more* beautiful. It was never just skin-deep.

RADICAL *thought*

Our goal was to treat the heart, uplift the soul, and help women shed the constraints of age or ailment, to feel more confident, and then pass that confidence on to someone else.

Longtime friend and radical sister on a mission, Maria Price shares her view of radical beauty: "The key to radical beauty is to respect yourself and to still see the beauty that you have inside and out. To not forget that it's there. But it starts by taking care of the inside so that beauty will resonate and appear on the outside. Be the best you can be no matter what your age. Develop yourself and make sure that you're taking advantage of the opportunities life puts in front of you. Say yes to life and the wonders that life has to offer. You have to be true to yourself no matter what because the only way to be happy is to be honest with yourself and go from there."

At the age of sixty-seven, Maria radiates beauty with her two seven-year-old twins! She took the *Radical Yes* seriously! At the end of the day, beauty is not just how you feel or how you look, but rather how you make the people around you *feel.*

Kindness is beautiful.

Grace is beautiful.

Radiance is beautiful.

Empathy is beautiful.

Intelligence is beautiful.

A sense of humor is beautiful.

Confidence is beautiful.

Sensitivity is beautiful.

Emotion is beautiful.

Authenticity is beautiful.

Generosity is beautiful.

Sharing is beautiful.

Love is beautiful.

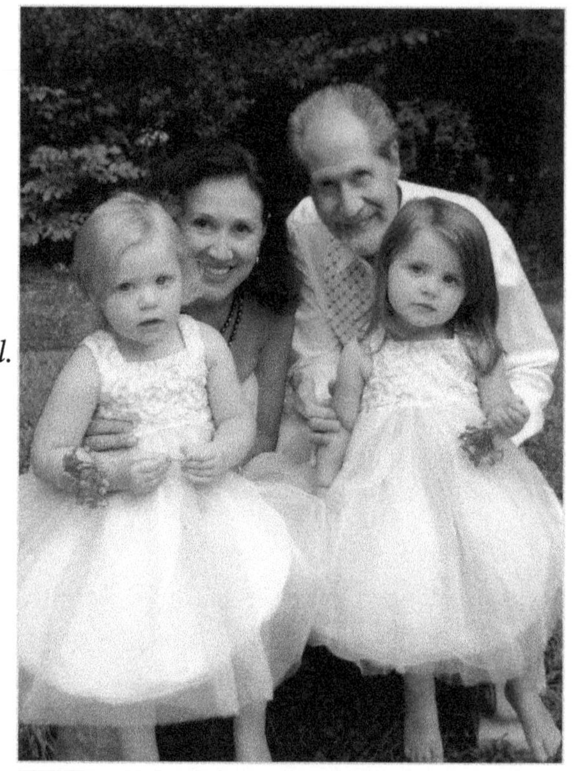

Maria Price, her husband Mike and their twin daughters Ali and Paige

Unforgettable moments are beautiful.

Enthusiasm is beautiful.

Vulnerability is beautiful.

What makes a woman beautiful? We can almost guarantee that it will not be the list you may find in those glossy magazines on the shelves. Around the world, people voiced their opinion that Radical beauty is making another's day, life, or spirit more beautiful so that they can then take that fullness in their heart and share it with the world. They act more beautiful. They see more beauty. They share that beauty. Then they are full enough to impart beauty onto another person. They are full enough to share with their children.

As Melanie Griffith says, "Radical beauty is enjoying the success and failures of your children. Being a parent is the hardest and most beautiful job in the world." When we are radically beautiful, we are full enough to share with our children, with our spouse, and with our significant other. We're full enough to share with people we know and those with whom we come into contact for the first time. That sense of fulfillment is contagious, and easy to catch."

JUST SHOW UP

In a traditional sense, so much of how advertising campaigns define beauty is based on looks. Mysterious eyes, a bright smile, long and wavy hair, high cheekbones, plump lips, proportionate facial features, a dainty and straight nose, and of course a fit and toned body. The media celebrates beautiful people and has informed us of their definition of beauty with endless pictures, photo shoots, videos, and other graphics. Articles and books are written about how to appear more beautiful and how to lose weight.

The American Society for Aesthetic Plastic Surgery reports that in 2013,

- Americans spent more than $12 billion on surgical and non-surgical procedures, the largest amount since the Great Recession in 2008. That is reflective of a 12 percent increase in the overall money spent.
- There were over 360,000 liposuction procedures performed in the United States, which surpassed breast augmentation as the most common procedure in 2013.
- Women had more than 10.3 million cosmetic procedures, 90.6 percent of the total.
- The number of cosmetic procedures for women increased over 471 percent from 1997.

"The numbers do not come as a surprise," states Jack Fisher, MD, president of ASAPS. "Technological advances, less-invasive procedures, greater accessibility are making aesthetic procedures, surgical and nonsurgical, far more attractive to the public at-large. Further, the rebounding economy is *encouraging people to start investing in themselves once again* [emphasis added]."

RADICAL *fact* | According to Canadian Skin Health Statistics, over $1 billion per year is spent on cosmetic treatments for the skin.[15]

But is this really the most fruitful investment? Sure, women across the country will tell you that these types of procedures make them appear and feel more beautiful. And there is value in the fact that they feel more beautiful. But we also strive to work toward progressing a different kind of investment, one that is focused on reinventing beauty and shifting its focus to how you feel, not just how you look.

Our society has created a definition of beauty that makes us all feel like not enough. You think, *I need more of that because without it I'm not going to be pretty enough.* You say, "I'm not going to be this enough. I'm not going to be that enough. It's never enough."

In the past, traditional beauty advertising and messaging have held us hostage to the faces of the unattainable, whether it is celebrities, eighteen-year-old models, or plastic surgeons promising overnight transformations. Women are now empowered, hungry, and demanding the truth about beauty and skincare. With the knowledge that the environment is playing an ominous role in what we ingest in our bodies, as well as what we put on our largest organ, our skin, the race is on to harness technology to extract the good and healing properties of nature while protecting us from the ever growing environmental aggressors.

Actress Emma Stone said, "My greatest hope for us as young women is to be kinder to ourselves so that we can be kinder to each other. To stop shaming ourselves and other people as 'too fat, too skinny, too short, too tall, too anything.' There is a sense that we are all 'too something' and we are all not enough. This is life. Our bodies change. Our lives change. Our hearts change."

Radical beauty means so much. It is more than skin-deep.

RADICAL BEAUTY MEANS SHOWING UP

How do you show up in the world?

That may be the singular most challenging question for us to answer. Showing up in an authentic manner is grounded in being vulnerable. When we show up, we often find that other people are willing to demonstrate that same authenticity. It is through that exchange of energy that the magic truly happens.

We know that the most beautiful people in the world are those who show up. They show up in unbelievably authentic and generous ways. They are kind, sincere, and willing to work to make others around them feel wonderful. Beauty is actually showing up in the world in a beautiful way, touching others and trying to make the world a better place, and making those around you have a better life. It screams beauty.

Liz: My very close girlfriend Goldie Hawn is beautiful. She exhibits multiple dimensions of beauty. When Goldie and I have traveled throughout the world together – Rome, Paris, London, Tahiti, Bahamas, and India to name part of the journey – Goldie led with laughter, and was steeped in spirituality and grace. Grace is beauty. We would be sitting in a restaurant in Rome trying to have a bite to eat, and there would be a line of people standing by us who wanted an autograph, a picture, a hello. After a while on our journey, I was amazed to see how she responded. I was personally exhausted. Exhausted by the nonstop intrusion. Wanting a moment to have a bite and not be interrupted. As I watched her respond, the word that came to mind again and again to me was GRACE. Goldie would smile and giggle and sign the napkin, take the photo, hug the stranger. No matter how many times, she was kind. That was beautiful. Radically beautiful.

Another story that comes to mind is when we were riding through Old Delhi, India, in a rickshaw, a carriage pulled by a bike, in wall-to-wall traffic, with elephants creating roadblocks. We were running late for our plane, but Goldie had promised an old friend a visit, no matter what it took. There we were, in the heat, traffic, and aggravation, and we decided to just give in to the absurdity of the moment and laugh. Just laugh. We eventually saw her friend, confined to a wheelchair in his modest home in India. She fulfilled her promise. That is radical beauty.

Melanie Griffith, our partner and lifetime friend, is one of the most generous spirits you will ever meet. Generous in heart, generous in friendship, generous in love, and willing to be vulnerable, authentic, and *there* for others. She supports the underdog. That is radical beauty.

One day I was in bed with the flu. Melanie called me and I told her how sick I felt. She said, "I make this incredible soup that will absolutely cure you. I swear!" I told her that was nice, but she lived in Hancock Park at the time and it would take her an hour or more to get to me and then, in traffic, even longer to get back home. She said, "I don't care, I am coming."

That's right, she drove three hours that day just to bring me her concoction to cure what ailed me. And when I told her that this was above and beyond, she told me it was nothing. She explained that she delivers her friend groceries at her house in the valley because she is in a wheelchair. That is radical beauty. The selfless act of loving another, giving to another, and showing up.

So, how do you show up?

You may not even know the answer. At times we don't know. But it is a question we ask of ourselves, discussing the answer often and trying to figure out how to improve that which we project to the world. But through these somewhat endless conversations, we figured out a few really important questions to ask:

- *Are you being something you are not?*
- *Are you being stingy with how you share with others?*
- *Are you being closed with your emotions?*
- *Are you giving your all to the world?*

RADICAL thought

The biggest room in the world is the room for improvement.

It is time for us as women to show up. As women, there comes a time when we have a sense of feeling depleted. We work so hard. We take care of our kids. We work to be great partners. We work to keep the house in order. We are doing all these things that really have nothing to do with how we feel. We're exhausted at the end of the day. We are running on fumes. There is literally nothing left.

RADICAL fact

Research shows that only 12 percent of women feel they are attractive.[16]

It is essential to find the time to recharge and reinvigorate our collective beauty so we can show up. As women, we have enormous responsibilities on so many levels. Many people call upon us and need our support and love. And it can be draining, which is completely normal. But we have to determine when we can no longer offer the world our innermost beauty. When that happens, we have a responsibility to renew that.

Have you ever noticed how you feel when you go out and take the time to be with some girlfriends and steal away an afternoon to laugh and let loose? After that time away, you'll likely feel as if you've got a new lease on life. You're able to laugh again, feel joy, and share and give and engage in the human spirit. Your magnetism, the light in your eyes, comes out. That's where beauty is.

- *Showing up is raw and electric.*
- *Showing up is sharing from your heart how you really feel.*
- *Showing up is being true to yourself so you can be true to everyone else.*
- *Showing up is being wholesome, selfless, and self-centered.*
- *Showing up radiates beauty and energy, and it draws people in.*
- *Showing up is beautiful.*

Only when we decide to show up in the world can we be the beauty for which the world thirsts. One of our parents' greatest qualities was showing up. Mom always showed up. She had a heart of gold, and it was always open to helping others. She never backed down from a challenge, and her willingness to selflessly be there for those in need was such an amazing character trait.

For our parents, beauty began where their skin ended. Their actions and behaviors taught us that beauty was not how you looked, but rather how people looked at you and how you made them feel.

- *Do they look at you with care and kindness?*
- *Do they look at you with love and emotion?*
- *Do they look at you with admiration and respect?*
- *Were they able to look at you at all?*

You have to be in the game of life to be seen, so show up. And do so in a radical way. Here is a list of beautiful acts that make you and the world more beautiful:

- Practice gratitude
- Remodel a loved one's house
- Pay for a stranger's food
- Take the time to listen to someone in need
- Bake a cake for someone you love
- Send off a handwritten card
- Compliment people often
- Hold the door for people

- Let cars go in front of you… even when there is traffic
- Give to charitable organizations
- Rescue an animal
- Listen more… talk less
- Cook meals for your loved ones
- Show emotion relentlessly
- Smile much more than you already do
- Give your children more time… not money
- Visit the elderly
- Recycle… and be conscious of the environment
- Tip better… especially when the service is great
- Don't ignore people… speak to them
- Surprise people more than you do
- Never underestimate the power of a hug
- Disconnect from technology for a few hours each week
- Be passionate about your life
- Don't give up so easily
- Manage adversity… don't let it manage you
- Spend more time immersed in nature and the outdoors

Beauty is everywhere. These are just a few examples of acts we have implemented to live radically beautiful lives. Each of these small yet meaningful actions helps to elevate both your life and the lives of those around you. Each of these small yet powerful steps will move you in the direction of beauty and love. You will begin to radiate and shine bright. That glow will become contagious, and you will find that you are a beacon of beauty – increasing smiles, enhancing warmth, and elevating lives.

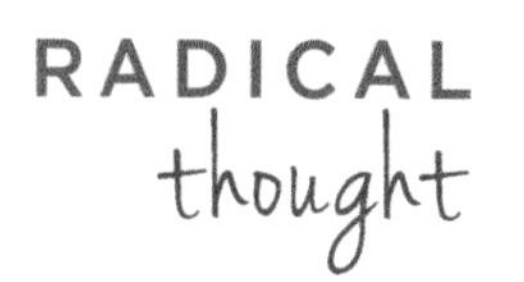

You have the power to awaken your inner beauty. Take time each day to remind yourself that you are beautiful, and you will start to feel more beautiful. Practice gratitude and see the difference inside and out.

RADICAL GRATITUDE

Rachel: Sometimes in life we take things for granted, including the ones closest to us. Family is very important in my life. My brother, sister, and I were raised to be best friends with one another from the time we were kids. Growing up on a farm created the perfect environment for bonding. Ever since Liz and I lived together in our twenties, my father always encouraged us to work together, knowing that we would always be there for each other. This is one of the greatest gifts that he ever gave us.

At that time, it sounded like one of my father's family talks that I'd heard a hundred times before. Even after being in business together for fifteen years, Liz and I are still best friends and business partners and are trying to change the world for the better in whatever way possible, whether big or small. My brother, who lives in Minnesota, was my best friend growing up, and he helped shape the person I am today.

Rich and I keep up with each other the best we can, though with our busy schedules, we don't connect as much as I would like. One of the most comforting things to know is that my brother and sister will be there for me if I need them. I always remind myself how lucky I am that we are all happy and healthy and that we have each other. We dealt with quite a bit growing up, seeing our father struggle with multiple sclerosis, and watching our mother contend with the pain of seeing her husband's health deteriorate month after month and year after year. After all of this, I figured the universe wouldn't put anything else on our plate to deal with, right? Wrong.

Early one Sunday morning, I received a phone call from my brother's wife, Patricia, saying that Rich had a seizure in the middle of the night and was in the hospital. My heart sank and I was in pure shock. She explained everything that happened to him, how long it lasted, and how the paramedics had to keep asking him what day it was and what his name was when he gained consciousness. My brother was completely disoriented. He had a difficult time answering their questions. She told me they had found a lesion on his brain.

I was on the verge of losing it when I realized that Patricia must have been at the brink of an emotional breakdown herself, and my sobbing would only make things worse. Panic set in. I began thinking of all the things that this could mean. I kept telling myself to remain positive. In just that moment, a wave of emotion came over me. I thought about not having my brother anymore. I reflected on our time growing up on the farm, playing football, lacrosse, fishing, fixing fences, chasing cows and pigs, and him torturing me by putting his smelly socks in my pillowcase and stapling my sheets together.

Years later, my kids and I spent time with him and his wife in Minnesota at Lake Ely. I wanted to give them the life experiences I had growing up. I remember running through fields, making up games using sticks and rocks. Those were the simple things in life that can easily slip away in the busy world I live in now. All of those experiences were priceless! As Rich lay in the hospital, I thought of never being able to share that with him again, and my kids missing out on precious time with their silly Uncle Rich.

Finally the doctors figured out it was a cavernomas, which are a cluster of blood vessels on the brain and *not* something as life threatening as a tumor. I was so grateful that it wasn't something fatal, but rather something that could be watched closely and dealt with by medication and surgery. The diagnosis was serious, but compared to the other options we would take it. As of this writing, Rich is forty-eight and now on seizure medication; he is still recovering.

When we spoke, I remembered again why he has been such a great influence in my life. He said, "I am so lucky that this wasn't fatal and that I have an amazing wife who has taken care of me in this moment of uncertainty and that my office is in close proximity to home so I can walk to work instead of drive." He always seems to see the glass half full at a time when he has every reason to complain about the negative.

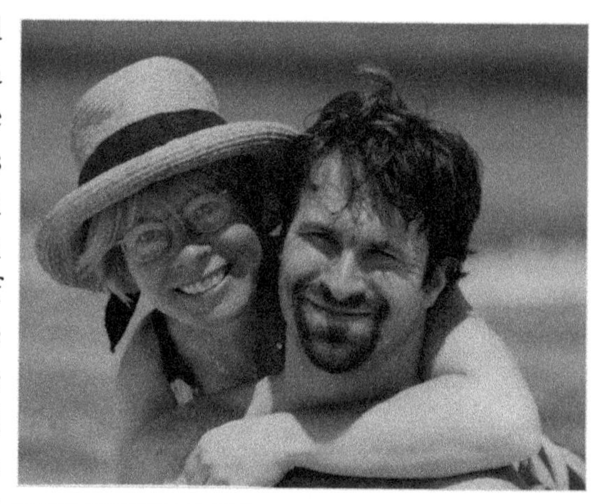

Our brother Richard Edlich and his wife Patricia

Reflecting on this moment brought me such an appreciation for my family and made me truly understand how fortunate I am to have the type of relationships with them that I do. I know many people who have estranged relationships with their family, and all I can do is encourage them to accept the differences, agree to disagree, and celebrate the relationship they can have today. It can be as simple as a call to check in, or as ambitious as a family vacation to create memories together, which are the pieces to the puzzle that make life beautiful.

Life is short. Yesterday can't be changed, and "Now" is all we have.

Beauty doesn't always shine through at first glance. But maybe that is part of the draw. Beauty is mysterious and requires investigation to be discovered. It is not always seen upon first glance. And therein lies the fun. As we travel through this crazy thing called life, we should all work and dedicate ourselves to give the gift of beauty and gratitude for our blessings, for the simple things before us that, if they were not there one day, would alter our lives forever. Our ability to make others feel beautiful is an enormous privilege and responsibility.

RADICAL *fact* | Writing down ten things a day that you are grateful for creates a sense of well-being and happiness. It lifts depression and gives you more of what you want.

Take this opportunity to stop reading and start listing what you are grateful for. Health, moments, a sunrise or sunset, your family, the ability to taste, hear, and see. The list is endless. Engage gratitude as your partner to create a life you love where you feel and look beautiful.

Liz: Every morning when I walk into the gym to see my trainer, Larry Willis, he will say, "Elizabeth, how are we today? How are you feeling?" I can feel myself moan at times. How am I feeling? It's 7 a.m., I didn't sleep enough, I am jet lagged AGAIN, gained weight on the road, my bones and muscles are aching, and he says, "How am I?" GRRRR…

Then he will say, "You are blessed! Look at this day. You are healthy and able to come to work out. Do you know how many people never got out of bed today? How many people do not have the legs or strength to lift themselves up? Every day is a blessing."

"Coach me, Coach!" I say. I know he is right, and I needed that reminder. Some days I get up and feel like there is an octopus on my face. I can't look at my world from a distance; rather, like in *Ghost Busters,* I got slimed by the day before with the negative and tiresome thoughts and forgot to celebrate my blessings.

Mind you, Larry is clearly beautiful on the outside. But it is his radical inspiration, gratitude, and loving nature that make him immensely beautiful. I take him with me on the road in my mind and hear his voice when I am weary. He says, "You got this, let's do one more for the haters and disbelievers, easy breezy cover girl, remember you make your money when no one is watching and the lights are off. Everything is easy when the stands are full and everyone is cheering. It's what you do behind the scenes when no one is looking that makes the difference. Successful people do what others won't." Spoken like a true professional football player. His words ring true to me, and I use them as a radical reminder.

Radical beauty is a gift from you to those around you. It is yours to give. Take that responsibility seriously. Because if we all do, we can collectively build a radically beautiful world.

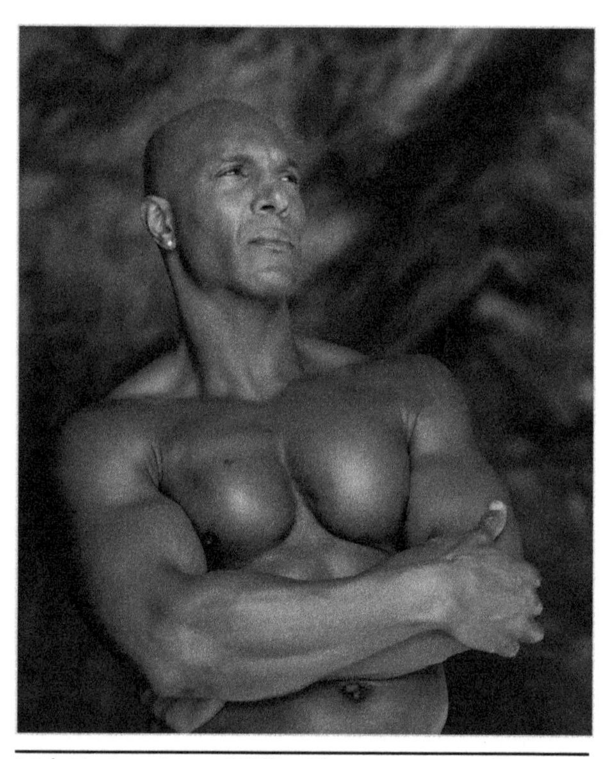

Liz's Trainer Larry Willis: Photo courtesy of Brian Pickett at Tenom Photos

Radical Recap:

When you find yourself questioning how radically beautiful you are, always remember that:

1. Beauty is something you give to others. Beauty is how you care for and treat those around you.
2. Studies have shown that writing down ten things a day that one is grateful for actually lifts people out of depression and makes them more beautiful.
3. Beauty comes from within. It resonates in your heart and soul and then is projected by how you behave and if you show up. Seize every opportunity you can to show up.

Chapter 15:
RADICAL LOVE

It can make us and it can break us, but regardless we search for it like the air we breathe.

It is a remarkable gift, probably the greatest gift we can give to one another.

It is much more valuable than any car, house, or piece of jewelry.

It is strong as granite but as fragile as a crystal vase.

It calls for nourishment to grow and develop, but once it matures it can often stand on its own.

Love.

Love is a lot of different things to a lot of different people, but more than anything it is connection.

That connection comes in an unbelievable spectrum of colors.

Love.

Love is truly without context, borders, restrictions, margins, and confines.

You can't contain it.

Love isn't something you could bottle even if you tried, and like sand, the more force you apply to holding onto it, the quicker it will escape from your grip and slip from your hands.

Paulo Coelho said, "When we love, we always strive to become better than we are. When we strive to become better than we are, everything around us becomes better too."

He said love makes the world a better place.

Beethoven reminded us that love is a "powerful emotion that has inspired countless artists to paint masterpieces, composers to write unforgettable music, and authors to pen bestselling novels."

He presumed that love inspires art.

Gandhi said, "Where there is love there is life."

He knew you couldn't have one without the other.

Lao Tzu knew that "being deeply loved by someone gives you strength, while loving someone deeply gives you courage."

He felt that love makes you more than you can be on your own. It elevates you.

Thoreau said, "There is no remedy for love but to love more."

Love is contagious and should spread.

But maybe it was Bob Marley's description of love that really brings us a vibrant perspective. He felt that when you are in love with someone: "Colors seem brighter and more brilliant. Laughter seems part of daily life where before it was infrequent or didn't exist at all. You think of this person on every occasion and in everything you do. Simple things bring them to mind like a pale blue sky, gentle wind, or even a storm cloud on the horizon. Life seems completely different, exciting, and worthwhile. Your only hope and security is in knowing that they are a part of your life."

That is the power of love.

Simply put, there is no substitution for love. It is one of most important ingredients within our prescription. There is nothing like it and no other piece can replace it. For Radical to work, radical needs love. It is one of the greatest gifts we can give to one another. Love is not always easy to define, but it is easy to see. You may not always be able to describe how it feels, but you know exactly when you are feeling it. At times you can smell it, you can touch it, and it arouses all of your senses like nothing else. Love is evolving and can change over time, but nonetheless it is a transformational energy that can heal and nourish both you and those around you.

So, *what is love?*

For as long as we can remember, love has always been a moving force in our lives. It has inspired, motivated, guided, blinded, uplifted, elevated, encouraged, enthused, excited, devastated, energized, and completely reshaped who we are, how we live, and what we feel. No other emotion has meant more to us than that simple four-letter word, *love*.

Defining love is a pretty overwhelming task to consider. But it is one we are going to take a shot at. Love is one of those really difficult topics because we all define it so differently. But we can agree that it is a necessity for each of us, as we all hope to eventually find unconditional and deep love.

Love manifests in so many different ways in this world: between friends, intimates, family members, God, animals; love of ideas, of principles, of possessions, of sports teams, of food, of coffee; love of sunsets, of sunrises, of destinations, of water and the beach, of the mountains or nature; love for kindness, for giving, for charity, for making a difference in the world. The people we love and the way in which we love is limitless. It lives without boundaries and can travel in any direction whatsoever.

We were recently talking about love with our girlfriend Dyan Cannon when she shared her own definition of it. She told us, "To me, God is love – capital L-O-V-E. Not the love that comes and goes. Not the love that doesn't keep its promises. Not the love that, in some instances, can turn to hatred. But a love that is constant and, in spite of anything we see, hear, feel or taste, that dominion that comes from that power is ever present in our lives. If I have been able to help anyone, it comes from that place of understanding and that type of love."

Similarly, Tracey Woodward shared that "radical love is knowing that the people who love you no matter what you do will always be there for you. That is why it is so important to love yourself. You are the most important person in your life. Without looking after yourself, you can't look after anyone else. It starts with you. Be kind and forgiving. Learn to move on. Love is everywhere – it knows no bounds."

THE EVOLUTION OF LOVE

From our perspective, the way we connect has a great influence on the way we love. Think about it. Centuries ago there was no cell phones, no Internet, and very limited mediums of communication. Love was limited, maybe in a good way, to that which happened when two people faced one another and looked into each other's eyes. That was the only way love could manifest itself—through presence and touch.

RADICAL *fact*

Studies show that we can relieve pain and stress simply by holding hands with a loved one.[17]

Fast forward to today. We love in lots of different ways. We call one another. We text one another. We send emails. We send pictures and videos. We can use technology to allow a grandparent to chat with his or her grandchild living in another country. We can effortlessly fold into the lives of one another with the Internet and the push of a few buttons. It is truly remarkable. But we might have traded that singular connection that occurs when you are looking at another person for the one that occurs when you are looking into your computer screen. Modernized love is convenient and accessible. It has increased our ability to connect and at the same time created a sense of disconnection because we can hide behind technology.

But at what cost?

As we mentioned above, we truly feel that love is imperative not only to our existence, but also to our happiness. How you are loved and how you give love is up to you. Giving and receiving love is the dance that brings love to life. Radical love starts with turning down the noise and allowing love to blossom and grow. Creating an environment in which love can flourish is key. So when we look at love through the ages, we feel confident in saying that to usher in a new era and protect the intensity and purity of love, we have to first build the environment for love to grow.

Rachel: I have two children, Forrest and Sophia. They have a special relationship. It's just this bond that sisters and brothers have. My son is protective of his little sister. Like any family, they have their moments when they don't get along and you wonder when they are going to be nice to one another, but overall they remain affectionate and you can see that the kind of relationship they have is genuine and full-hearted. They care about the little things like recognizing what each other likes and doesn't like. It's the little things that matter in how they show each other love.

When Sophia was born, Forrest was very hands-on with her and held her and helped to take care of her. He was a great big brother in that capacity. As she grew, she started to learn from him. She actually imitates him and has this great sense of humor that really engages her brother, so they're constantly being silly and playing together.

On numerous occasions, I remind them how lucky they are to have one another. Of course, they look at me like I am crazy and continue to get under each other's skin. Good old sibling love. Growing up, I remember doing that to my brother like it was yesterday.

Take dinnertime at my house. Family dinners are very important to us. It is a time to come together and connect with each other about our day. It's where we have the opportunity to create the environment for love to grow. One particular week was plagued with bickering between them. After two days of this relentless interchange, they saw no reason to change direction and it continued throughout dinner as well.

Exhausted from trying to make them stop, I decided to take a different approach, a heart-opening approach. I came from love. I asked each person at the table to share what they loved about each other. Forrest and Sophia quickly looked at each other with sweet smiles. I could see the wheels were turning to create a list of what they loved about each person at the table. Everybody had to go around and tell one another what was special about their brother, sister, mother, and father. That simple act of sharing with one another and being able to verbalize love with our children was extremely meaningful.

Saying what you love about someone out loud while looking at that person opens your heart up to love. Sharing knowledge as to why each person is so special is a gift. I can tell you that the energy shift at the table was instantaneous.

Forrest started by sharing why he loved Sophia. At this time, Forrest was twelve and not overly expressive. The loving words he shared about each person there was a huge deal for me. As he spoke, you could feel the love radiate around the table. Sophia, on the other hand, who was six, couldn't stop sharing what she loved about each person. In fact, she wanted another turn to go around! It started with loving Forrest's smile and how he let her play in his room. Small things, but at that age, small things are what represent the love they have for one another. You could see how her sharing created warmth, love, sweet smiles, laughter, and hugs. The tone of our dinner and house completely changed. After that they played lovingly together.

Verbally saying to someone why you love them shifts the energy and creates an open and receptive heart. It is now our ritual once a month at our dinner table to show love and remind us how lucky we are to have each other every day. There are no rules. There are no requirements. My kids can do it in any fashion they choose. However it is done, and what remains is the gift of love and an environment that nurtures love, allowing it to blossom in all its glory.

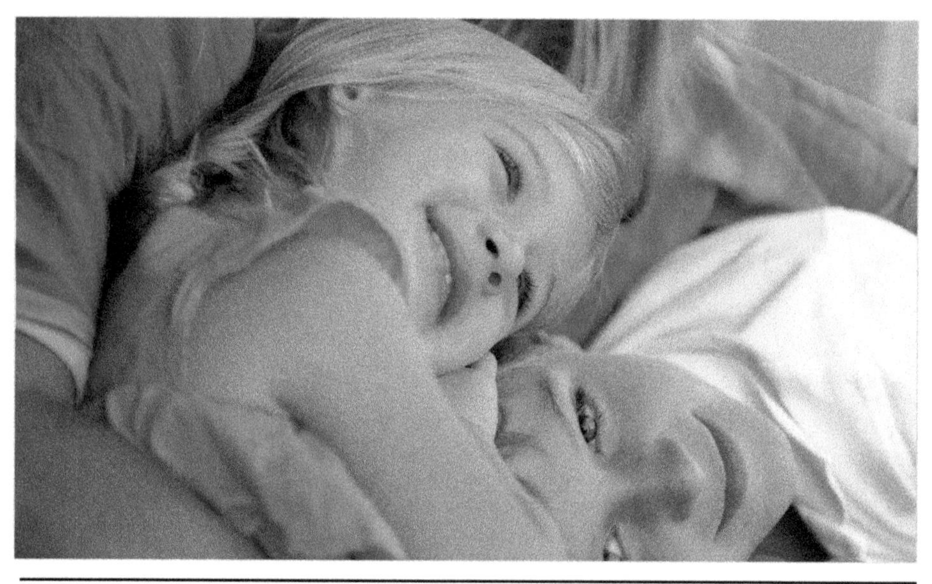

Rachel's kids Sophia and Forrest

Love evolves.

Whether we are growing and changing as children or growing and changing as adults, it requires the interest and dedication to learn and relearn, at each phase in life, what love looks like to us and what it looks like to those around us. Many times what was important to us in our twenties or thirties is no longer our first priority. So while the core heartbeat of love remains over time, how it beats and what rhythm it adopts is important to its survival.

Teach your friends, your family, your loved ones, and others in your life that love is the exchange of emotion. It is energy that is generated and then passed from one person to another. Because giving that energy to another is one of the greatest gifts you have at your disposal.

THE SCIENCE OF LOVE

Love is a powerful emotion. So much so that there is actual science supporting how you fall in love. That's right – as you progress in your feelings, emotions, and attractions for someone, your body releases chemicals that create that warm and fuzzy feelings on the inside. Think about how you feel when you are attracted to someone or begin to fall in love. You can literally feel a change in your physical makeup, and it spreads throughout your body.

RADICAL *fact*

Ever experienced butterflies in your stomach when falling in love? Well, turns out it is actually adrenaline flooding your body.[18]

Radical love occurs the same way. It is intense and is the result of the release and interaction of these chemicals, just more of them. It is that connection and energy that helps to introduce these powerful chemicals, which then create some pretty lasting effects.

For example:

- *When you fall in love, you'll find decreased levels of serotonin, which result in erratic behavior. That is why you are nervous and anxious around people to whom you are initially attracted.*
- *As you become attracted to someone, you'll find an increase of your cortisol levels, which is often released as a response to a stressful situation.*
- *Dopamine starts pouring into your brain, creating that awesome feeling of euphoria, sleeplessness, loss of appetite, and a rush of creativity and inspiration.*
- *Dopamine also spikes in moments of extreme intensity, like kissing or other physical contact.*

- *Epinephrine and norepinephrine also increase, causing your heart to beat faster, and introduce more oxygen into your brain.*
- *The "love hormone" or oxytocin is often triggered by kissing.*

It is amazing to consider that the emotion or feeling of love can create all of these physical changes in your body. And that is partially why love is so radical. Very few emotions result in such immediate and substantial modifications to your physiological makeup. The point is that when you feel clammy hands, your heart beating out of your chest, that sensation of euphoria, and you just can't fall asleep, it is possible that you are falling in love. But falling in love is just one part of radical love. And through understanding love, you'll be better positioned to give it back to those around you.

THE FIVE LOVE LANGUAGES ARE:

So how do you identify with love?

That is a question we should each constantly ask ourselves. If not, it is easy to find ourselves and our loved ones feeling unloved and frustrated. Remember, knowledge is power. And knowing our tendencies and the way we love is crucial when introducing love into our lives. And the more power we have over our life and our ability to manifest love and happiness, the higher quality of life we will experience.

Knowing that love manifests in so many different ways gives us an exciting and uplifting opportunity to make it our own. We all feel and understand love differently. We will have a much higher probability of choosing the right partner when we understand what makes us tick and what makes our partner tick.

A phenomenal tool that we keep referring to is *The Five Love Languages,* a New York Times bestseller by Dr. Gary Chapman. In his book, he outlines the five ways in which people express and experience love. And when you determine what your primary love language is, half the battle is won.

These include:

1. **Words of Affirmation:** This love language uses words to affirm other people (compliments and acknowledgments).

2. **Acts of Service:** For these people, actions speak louder than words (you respond to people doing something for you).
3. **Receiving Gifts:** For some people, what makes them feel most loved is to receive a gift.
4. **Quality Time:** This language is all about giving the other person your undivided attention.
5. **Physical Touch:** To this person, nothing speaks more deeply than physical touch.

Identifying and understanding how you best receive love and express it gives you clarity about what you want and how you want it. Remember that unless you are clear on what you want and how you want it, it is impossible to ask for it or recognize it. This clarity is gold to a person who wants love and fulfillment.

RADICAL *thought*

Want to increase your happiness? Tell the people you love how thankful and grateful you are to have them in your life.

Whether it is a romantic relationship, friendship, or family member, people identify with love in these five different ways. Some people feel affirmation is the most expressive sense of love. Others need quality time or even physical touch to feel loved. If your partner requires you to "do something" to feel loved, and you are constantly "offering affirmation or compliments," he may feel unfulfilled, even though you are putting forth the effort to show him how much you care.

Thoughtful love is often the best kind. The reason why? Because it hits home with the people you are thinking about. We are pre-wired to love and be loved. But we all interpret and appreciate love in ways specific to the fabric of our heart and souls. And that is why understanding what type of love you want and what means the most to you, and then working to learn how others need to be loved, brings fulfillment and happiness. Knowing this can change your love life radically.

So understanding that there are different ways to show your love is pivotal to building radical love. Radical love is the type of love that connects people and builds energy. Love can be engaged or expressed with and for a lot of different people and in a lot of different categories in life. Radical love is love with meaning. Taking love past normal limitations by using the five languages of love to identify how to love yourself and others at a remarkable level is a gift.

Take the time to study the five different love languages and how they are expressed in real life. Then study how you like to be loved and project that to the world. Finally, by asking about others' love languages, you will learn how to give them exactly what they want – love in the way they can feel it and experience it.

RADICAL LOVE STARTS WITH YOU

Rachel: Radical living is steeped in giving back to others. It embraces the point of view that going above and beyond and touching someone's life in even the smallest way can make a difference. The one area of radical living that I seem to overlook is self. To be completely honest, self-care seems to happen only when I get so maxed out on everything and everyone needing something from me that I ask myself, "What about me?" It has happened to me again and again. There are times when I open my eyes and say, "Why am I so tired, uninspired, and feeling this emptiness? Why does this feel so familiar?" Work, kids, marriage, friends, and family seem to take up every free moment, and I forget to squeeze out some time for the things that bring me personal joy.

As usual, I didn't stop to recognize that I needed to take care of myself until the perfect storm hit on a trip to a hot springs hotel. Fortunately, the stars were in alignment for me to experience this much-needed self-care. I had someone to watch the kids for the night, my friends weren't available to join me, and my husband was unexpectedly out of town.

This trip was supposed to be for my husband and me, but now he couldn't make it. So I made the decision to take some time for myself. A part of me thought it would be best to cancel and save the money. It would also give me some time to catch up on work and hang with the kids. But the other part of me said, "Why don't you treat yourself to some R&R? You deserve it."

The next thing to enter my mind was whether or not I would be lonely, bored, and unsettled with no distractions. I forgot what it was like to have nothing to do and just be in the moment. So I made the effort to practice what I preach and embrace the opportunity to let this adventure with myself unfold, and say the *Radical Yes* to self.

When I arrived in Palm Desert, I decided to turn off my phone, pretend as if there were no TV, and be open to what was around me.

The voices in my head didn't want to give me a vacation. They started the chatter of how I was going to eat lunch and dinner alone. *Will people be staring at me in the restaurant? I've seen others do it, but I've never done it myself.* By then, my hunger took over. I ordered what I wanted, read a magazine, and took in others' conversations. I had nobody to look after but myself. Thinking that I would soon become bored at dinner alone, I decided to enjoy every bite like my mom does. She's the slowest eater I've ever known, and I'm the exact opposite. For the first time in a long time, I didn't feel rushed. I savored every bite. How wonderful it was!

I left the restaurant and hurried back to my hotel room. In my mind I was already three steps ahead of myself, tucked in bed, and done with the day. Why do I do that? I heard a little voice inside me say, *be present in the moment, Rachel.* Immediately I stopped. I took a deep breath and told myself to slow down because I wasn't in a rush to be anywhere. So I found a comfy chair and gazed at the pure beauty of the night. *Slow down* should be a phrase I repeat over and over to stop my mind from jumping ahead.

Sometimes I go through life forgetting to take in the crescent moon, the stars shining brightly, the beauty of a warm summer evening, and the wind dancing through the trees.

Through this experience, I realized that by running on empty and not taking time for myself, I'm less able to fulfill my responsibilities in making a difference in my work, family, and friendships. Taking care of myself makes me a better mother, wife, and advocate on this Radical Skincare mission.

I believe that we all strive to be the best we can be, but by ignoring our need to take care of ourselves, we are doing a huge disservice to ourselves and others. So don't wait for the perfect storm or breakdown before you take that precious time out for you. Make it a self-imposed ritual to say "YES" to your radical self and love yourself radically.

A Radical Reminder:

Embrace:

1. The love you have for yourself

2. The love you have for others

The love you have for yourself encompasses things like:

- *How you treat yourself*
- *How you view your mind and body*
- *How you work to grow and develop internally and externally*
- *How you talk about yourself and to yourself*
- *How you allow others to love you*
- *How you express and project yourself to the world*

The manner in which you demonstrate each of these pivotal pieces is ultimately indicative of the love that you have for yourself. The more we love ourselves, the more we can allow others to love us. As we develop our self-love and grow personally, we can then take great strides in developing this same love for those around us, which leads us to the love we have for others.

The love we have for others touches on things like:

- *How we make people feel about themselves*
- *How we treat people we know and those we don't*
- *How we elevate and uplift people*
- *How we help others, and the difference we make in their lives*
- *How we deliver on that trust or not*

Liz: About three years ago, while we were in the beginning stages of building our new personal passion, Radical Skincare, we also had to manage our other existing business.

And the day came when a very profitable opportunity arose. One that would for most feel like a blessing, but for us felt like a curse. A company made an offer to purchase one of our businesses. The one condition for the purchase was that they wanted Rachel to go with the acquiring company.

They offered a substantial buyout as well as a pretty nice package for Rachel to remain. She would have received enormous financial stability at a time when it would have been more than welcomed.

Radical Skincare was growing but was costing us a lot, and it was our labor of passion and love, not monetary gain that was keeping us going. Remember, we had never intended to make it a business. It was a passion and purpose project that took on a life of its own.

As we entertained this lucrative offer, I told Rachel that she should do what was best for her family. As I bit my lower lip, wanting to say the right and generous thing, I knew in my heart that my Radical Skincare journey would not be long lived as a solo adventure. To me, it was our love that made the company so special, and doing it together empowered us both. That was the payoff. The minute the sister journey went away, the minute it wasn't an "us" being able to share our life journey together, the minute that love and connection was potentially gone from the day-to-day would be the minute the adventure would end for me. I was ready to sell our baby business, Radical Skincare, if Rachel left, and I told my new investor partner so.

Rachel: What a challenging moment this was for me. Do I go with the company where we could all receive huge financial gain from a sale? The problem was that I didn't want to work for this company. It wasn't where my passion was. But I felt like everyone was counting on me since I was the one condition for the deal to go through. So after many sleepless nights and long talks with Liz, I turned down the substantial salary and $1.7 million buyout for me personally. Yep... you read that correctly. I walked away from it.

Why?

I did it because I knew that Radical Skincare was radical love, and not being able to share the journey with my sister left me feeling empty inside. Also, I knew that my life with this new company would never be on my own terms. It would pull me away from my children, and it would call for a substantial amount of my time working with people who saw the world differently than me. Different values altogether.

It was my love for Liz and our love for working together that made me say, "Okay, I will go do anything, I will work day and night on this journey no matter how difficult it can be. It will all work out because we can do it together as a family. And we can do it on our own terms." That, to me, was a very clear example in our lives where there was love, there was passion, and there was purpose. It was radical.

It was a strange dynamic. With over a million dollars on the table, we both felt nothing but depression at the thought of taking it and leaving our radical dream.

- *Depression in breaking up Radical Skincare*
- *Depression in working with people who didn't have the same values*
- *Depression in not working with each other*

Radical Skincare has always been something so much greater than a skincare line. Radical Skincare has always been radical love. Radical love between two sisters. Between friends. Between family. Between colleagues. As we built our company, we were a tornado, sucking in all of the people we love and finding a way for them to play a role, whether it was business advice or guinea pigs for tour products or marketing experts or any one of a million other roles. Radical Skincare taught us how to love radically. And it gave us many of the tools and resources to share our radical love with you.

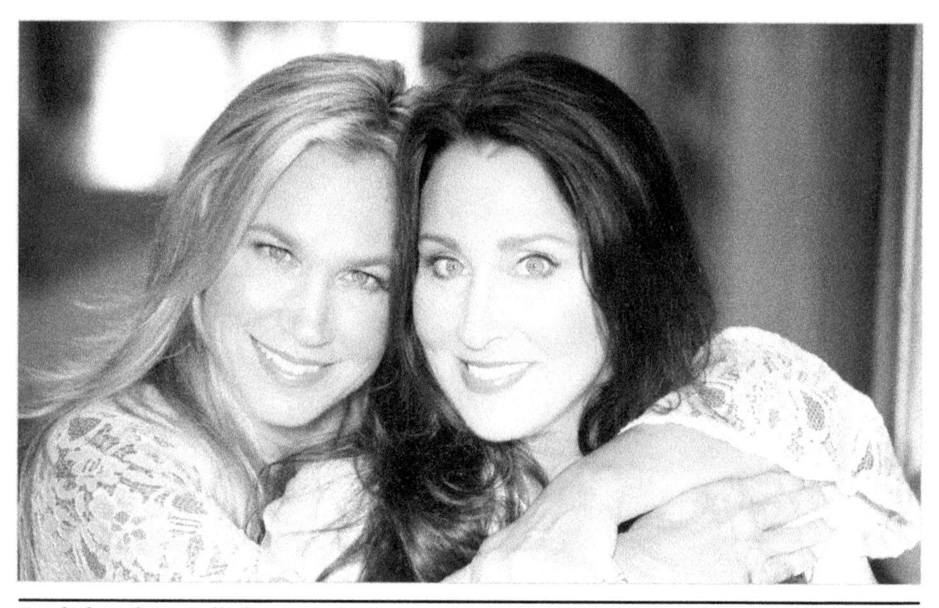

Rachel and Liz Edlich

We believe we are all born destined for love. It is a fundamental human need. We all thirst for it. Radical love is connection. It is the exchange of energy at an increasingly high frequency. It is understanding one another so we can love harder and with more meaning. Radical Skincare was born from radical love. It was the love between us that helped us build the foundation for the business. It is our commitment to have a life of purpose that has us share this with you. Our story, our lessons, and our life-changing skincare.

Radical Recap:

To invite Radical Love into your life, always remember that:

1. Few things in life are more important than love. Love is a powerful emotion that can move mountains and change lives.

2. Love constantly evolves. It is different at different ages and stages of our lives.

3. Knowing how you feel love and how another interprets and feels love gives you the ability to create fulfilling and loving relationships. Use the power of love to inspire you.

4. Finally, the more we love ourselves, the more we can allow others to love us. Love yourself first, and welcome in everyone else in the process.

Chapter 16:
RADICAL GIVING

I*t has the ability to cure hunger.*

It can eliminate the poverty we see on the street corners of our cities.

It can help to put a roof over a child's head.

While it makes the giver feel good, it makes the receiver feel treasured.

Giving. Charity. Philanthropy. Love.

It literally keeps the world going.

Radical giving means making a difference by being the difference.

As sisters, we heard this phrase all the time. That was the mantra our father gave us growing up. To make a difference you must be a difference. Being a difference is showing up to make an impact. When you wake up, how are you going to make an impact? It doesn't have to be the biggest footprint in the world. It could simply be a series of small thumbprints. But the inevitable goal is to do enough good to leave a legacy behind. To make a difference in the lives of others through gratitude, kindness, and love, while remembering that we are all in this together.

Rachel: For me, it's very clear-cut. You make a difference by helping others. Everybody has the ability to do that. The difference can be a series of small things. They do not have to be enormously large. Every morning I wake up and make my kids lunch before ushering them off to school. I always make sure they are happy, well-fed, and have all the tools they need to prepare for a positive day. It is a small difference, but it makes all the difference in their ability to be educated.

Liz: Spending five dollars at 5 a.m. was the best money I spent all day. As I was walking through the airport that morning, I realized I had already been up for almost three hours. What was the point of sleeping when I had to catch an early flight? I decided to grab a snack while I waited to board the plane. I wandered over to a kiosk where I spotted a bag of potato chips (which I rarely eat) calling my name. Calories before 6 a.m. didn't count, did they?

I walked up to the stand where there was a man and a young woman working. The girl hardly noticed me and continued to frantically count the money in her drawer. She had a scowl on her face. As I inquired about the unhappy face, she seemed overwhelmed with panic and didn't respond. On her second count of the cash drawer, I overheard the man behind her say, "Maybe the five dollars ended up in your pocket."

The reason for the scowl on her face became clear as day. At that moment, I decided to speak my piece and told him the money was not in her pocket. I asked her if she needed money to cover the drawer. She looked up at me in disbelief and said, "Yes." So I offered up a five-dollar bill I had in my wallet. She took the money and put it in the drawer, rang up my order, and graciously thanked me.

After I could see the relief in her eyes, I suggested we both smile and use this experience to brighten someone else's day. She looked at me with an ear-to-ear grin and said, "Have a great day and a great flight!" I thanked her, and while I made my way to catch my flight, I couldn't help but think how five dollars lifted her load a little bit.

Such a small bit of kindness that potentially saved this young girl her job. Maybe it was a job she needed to support her family or pay for college.

Who knows?

But that small act could have monumental impact.

RADICAL *fact*

According to an article in Forbes magazine, giving to others not only makes you feel good, but also strengthens your heart, literally![19]

How can we be that contribution? It shows up differently every day. It's not always going to be the same thing. How can each of us make that difference? How can we show up in the lives of others? When it comes to radical giving, all you have to do is show up. The world thirsts for the reciprocity of giving. It is not only needed, it is imperative for our continued growth, development, and evolution.

THE ROOTS OF RADICAL GIVING

For us, radical giving started at a young age. Our parents instilled that attitude into the fabric of our DNA, and it truly shined through. So much so that it was hard for them to punish us when we acted like a modern-day Robin Hood. Growing up, we were rather close with our neighbors. But there were few we loved more than Ms. Clemens. We lived on a farm in Charlottesville, Virginia. She owned a trailer across the street from our long gravel driveway. We always enjoyed spending time with her. She was quite elderly and always welcomed us in, three little rug rats with endless energy.

Ms. Clemens and her husband had no running water or plumbing. They struggled monthly to pay their bills. But that didn't stop her from always giving us a small treasure when we left her house. She was truly the trophy girl for radical giving. After visiting, she would always give us a party favor in the form of a small horse figurine. She had a large collection of them and was always willing to share with us. Great excitement surrounded our almost daily trips to Ms. Clemens's house. She had a way of making us feel wanted and loved. It was her radical giving, even on a small level, that made us, as little girls, feel so special.

So naturally we wanted to return the favor.

Liz: Even as a young girl, I loved design and decorating. I spent hours moving furniture around in my room and even ventured into the other rooms of the house in an effort to surprise our mother. So when I noticed that Ms. Clemens's trailer walls were bare and empty, I decided to emulate my mother's giving spirit; I knew I had to do something. Knowing that Ms. Clemens was really in need, I used to put our leftovers from dinner on a plate, and I would walk them up to her house. She would greet me with a toothless grin, holding her cup of moonshine, and devour my goodies.

So this particular day, I decided maybe I should help her decorate. But since I didn't have any money, the only thing I could do was to take some of Mom's paintings and pictures off of our walls and carry them over to Ms. Clemens's trailer. When I made it there, I hung them on her wall and smiled with a great sense of accomplishment. Well, that ended quickly when I returned home. While I was gone, my mother returned from the store, only to find her once-filled walls partially empty. She must have thought that we were robbed.

Mom looked at me and said, "Uh, darling, where is that painting of the flowers?"

"Oh, I gave it to Mrs. Clemens."

"You what?" she said."My friend gave me that. That was a gift to me. You can't take things that don't belong to you."

I said, "Yeah, I can. She doesn't have anything on her walls, and we have plenty on our walls, and you always taught me to give to those in need."

In that moment I realized two things. The first was that I had gone too far. The second was that even in her frustration of finding out I had just given away an irreplaceable picture, Mom still remained proud of my giving spirit. She knew then that I was learning at a young age to be a radical giver.

Giving is in all of our roots. Gratitude is a sense of being. It gives you the exciting opportunity to have perspective and take note of your blessings. It's how you walk through life when you're taking into account all the positive things around you. The fact that you can physically walk through life at all is a reason to be grateful. The fact that you can get up in the morning and have the legs and strength to do so.

Because of our father's illness and our mother's dementia, we had quite a bit of degenerative diseases in the family and experienced these difficult situations in a close-up and personal manner. One of the most beautiful acts of giving is the story of Laura Makowski who we offered an internship when we met her in Germany. She said that she had a dream of working in America. So we said the Radical Yes and offered to fly her to Los Angeles and told her that she could live with our mother and use her car and work for Radical. We believed at the time that we were giving to Laura and mentoring her, but it turned out that she was the gift.

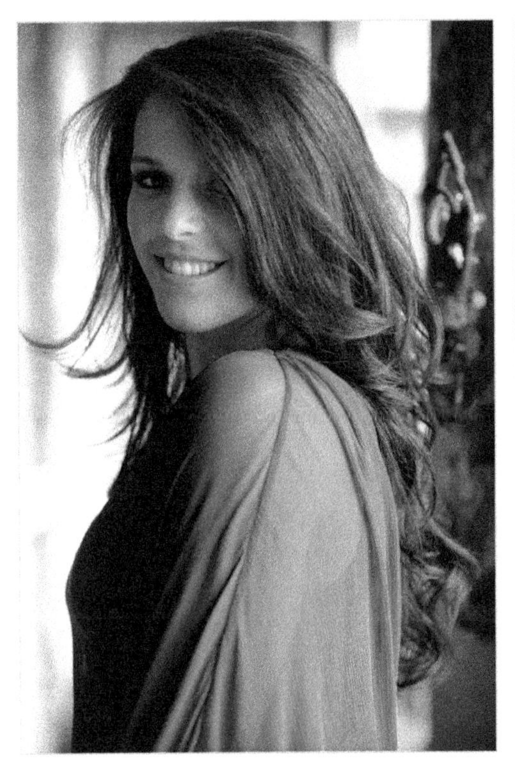

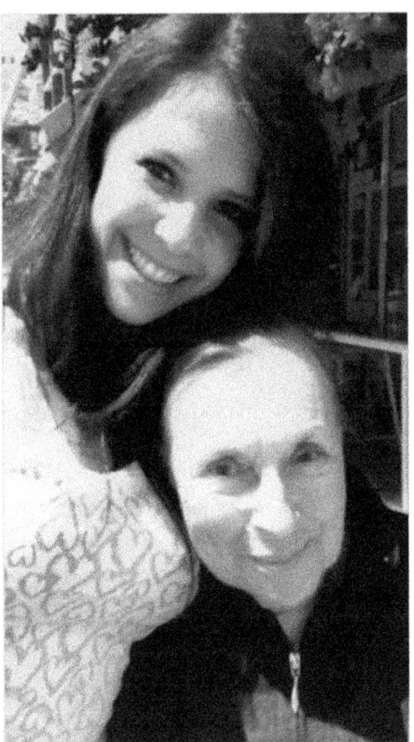

Our Mom Carol Edlich's Caretaker and friend Laura Makowski

For more about Liz and Rachel's mom visit her caretaker Laura Makowski's Living Portrait on the Radical Living section of our website www.radicalskincare.com/living.

Living with our mother, Laura uncovered the depression in her days that she hid so well during our visits. Her anxiety and fear of losing her memory that caused her to write daily an account of every hour, what she ate, what she drank, what medication she took, and who she spoke to. We had no idea how much her illness had progressed. Laura coached our family through moving our mother into an assisted living situation and helped us learn how to better communicate with her and accept her in her new state of cognition. Laura's giving nature and commitment to transition our mom and the family into a new life after dementia was one of the greatest gifts that we have ever received. And to think that we thought we were the ones giving her the gift.

These experiences can give you a sense of perspective and push you to do all you can to help those in need. Take time every day to just look around.

There is so much opportunity to give if you just open your eyes. The gift in the end will be yours to cherish.

Flex your giving muscle.

If you're walking, you could open the door for somebody so that they walk through first. If you can help someone across the street, seize the opportunity! Start to look for opportunities to give. Even start to knock off the small ones because, as you do that, then you become even more aware of how you can give. You create muscle memory and train your giving muscles to always be ready to act on an opportunity for kindness.

As Caroline Hirons says, "Giving is crucial. It makes you feel good. If you cannot do it financially, you can give of your time. My kids know that nothing new is coming in the house until they go through all that they have and give things away."

RADICAL thought | If you are having a bad day, the best thing you can do is help someone else in need.

You can then become a soldier in search of opportunities to give. Just start saying yes. Say that *Radical Yes* to giving. Then it becomes second nature. As you reflect back on your day, you will recognize the opportunities that were before you and celebrate that you seized them all.

Our brother Richard takes time every week to mentor kids in his community. He does this even though he is battling serious health issues. He supports charities and always roots for the underdog. Richard is the one person that can bring us back to our core. Growing up, he was not a particularly emotional person and a bit of a rebel, but Rich is very grounded. His essence is so clear and sensitive that it can be unnerving. We are constantly amazed at the quality of life that he maintains to create heartfelt moments of tradition, simplicity, and an uncomplicated wonder through his giving nature. Since he is part of the family, it makes sense that he shares a similar view of radical giving.

Rich says, "To me, radical is not about taking monstrous steps in changing the world; it is more about taking one small step. We've got to be okay with taking the smaller steps and trusting it, and knowing that some things can't be accomplished overnight. Change takes time, but it starts with giving and truly taking a stand to live. Where do we make that difference? When we're in a place of calm, when we're in a place of reflection, and when we're in a place of support and love – that's where the changes occur. It allows us to begin the process of giving. We have to give quietly and consciously and get people to participate in their own lives so that they can contribute as well. That's where the small steps occur. And for many people, those small steps, and that giving, can make a big difference."

We often traverse life looking down. Down at our phones, down at our laptops, and down at the ground in an effort to be seemingly connected and efficient. But the reality is that we don't connect with those who are in front of us. We are too busy or scared. If we actually just put our heads up and looked around, we may say, gosh, there are some opportunities to give and to support another human being.

We were lucky to be raised to look up, look around, and find the occasions where we can selflessly make a difference in the life of another person, even if it means taking our mom's favorite flower painting off the wall and giving it to another.

BE THE LAST PERSON ON THE PLANE

Giving is such a gentle yet powerful word. We love the way it sounds, the way it elegantly rolls off the tongue. Giving is powerful enough to hold its own space and place, and the act of being kind creates an overall sense of well-being. You feel better, look better, and are physically healthier when engaging in an act of kindness. Be it to a person or an animal, the act itself will empower and energize you.

Our mother is one of the kindest people we know. She is an angel, and we would often say to ourselves, "If only we could be as giving as our mother." She is the one that will laugh and have conversations with everyone she meets. She will want to adopt the man washing her car or bagging her groceries, the child giggling in the park, even the dog or cat that needs a home. That's why we had eight dachshunds, two cats, two goats, cows, horses, and pigs as pets growing up. She took radical giving to a whole new level. She is the difference the world deserves.

Liz: Recently, I was at JFK airport heading out on one of my many business trips. Standing in the security line, I began preparing my bags for the

X-ray machine and readied myself for the never-ending scrutiny of my belongings. I noticed there was a bag delivered to the conveyer belt with a little blue ribbon tied to it to make it easier to recognize. It reminded me of what my mom would do. Curious as to whom the owner of this lonely bag was, I looked around and saw an older lady, a bit hunched over like Mom, rifling through her wallet and papers to present her ID and tickets to the security officer. As the line grew behind her, I thought I might help her through the new travel procedures. After all, I would hope that someone would do the same for my mom.

I went over to her and suggested that we do this together. She explained that she was eighty years old and going down to Florida to see her son. She told me that she was too old to do this and that she was unsure as to what she was supposed to do to get through security. I told her, "You are not old, you're wise, and compared to all of the things you have done in your eighty years, this is going to be a piece of cake!"

So we removed her shoes and put all of her things through the X-ray machine. As luck would have it, they pulled her bag and searched it. After helping her put everything back into its place, I asked her where her gate was. Her gate was in the opposite direction of mine, but I wanted to make sure she got there safely. My flight was leaving in twenty-five minutes, but I was used to being the last one on the plane. As we proceeded toward her gate, she informed me that her flight didn't leave for five hours; she just wanted to make sure she was there in time. Then she looked up at me and asked if I worked for the airlines.

"No," I said, smiling. "Maybe just for you today."

"Well, you are like an angel and you're so pretty," she said. "You could be on TV or something."

We reached her gate and she settled in. I thanked her for allowing me to help and gave her a hug as I quickly ran to my gate, and of course I was the last person on the plane.

Finally, I was earning my wings and taking a couple of small steps to be kind like my mom. It was a rewarding feeling to see the older woman's appreciation and know that she was safely where she needed to be. As I ran to catch my flight, I could barely hold back my tears. I was unbelievably

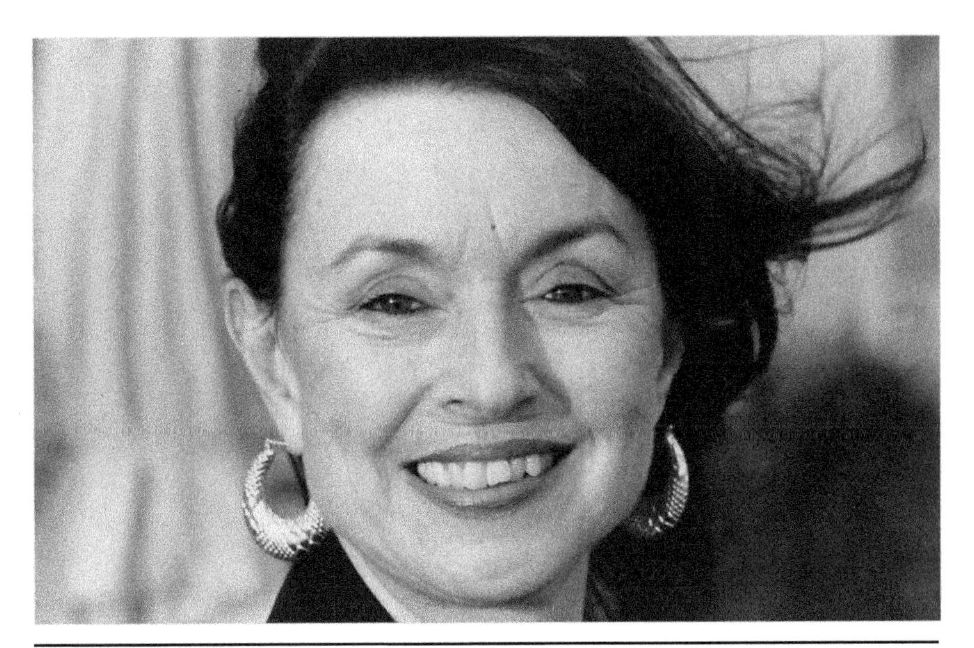

Our mom, Carol Edlich who was always kind to others

touched by the power of taking a moment to be there for another person and do the simplest of things. I carried her smiling eyes around with me in my thoughts and it lifted my spirits, giving me a sense of peace. I had all the reasons in the world not to help her: the lines, the hassles, the flight, she wasn't my mom or my problem. I was busy, had phone calls to make, and so many seemingly important things to do. As it turned out, those moments walking through the airport with her ended up being the most important thing I did that day, and easily the most rewarding.

In life, we always have the opportunity to be the last person on the plane and to sacrifice time or energy or money to make a difference in the lives of others. It is often that act of giving that positions us to be the receiver of so much more. Ralph Waldo Emerson said, "The purpose of life is not to be happy. It is to be useful, to be honorable, to be compassionate, to have it make some difference that you have lived and lived well." Say yes to the chance of leaving a thumbprint on other's lives.

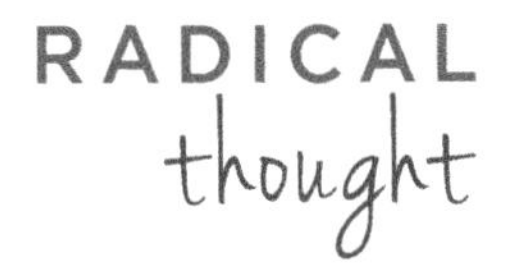

Living a radical life helps you share what you have learned with others and teaches you to be in the present moment and enjoy the journey. Do not stay stuck in yesterday or live in tomorrow. Remember, we only have today.

Don't allow these timeless moments to pass you by. The gifts you receive in return will far exceed your investment. The return will be amazing. And that return is not just personal. It inspires others to do more. Our mother instilled in us a sense of compassion and kindness that should be shared. That was her gift to us. And we feel strongly that we have a duty and a responsibility to pass that along to the world.

THE JOURNEY OF GIVING

You never know where your giving will lead you or exactly what it will accomplish, but one thing for sure is that you'll feel great doing it. This appears to be a selfless venture, but when you understand the payoff it can actually be seen as a self-empowering venture, because the return you will reap is huge. The time, the energy, and the money will always pale in comparison to the unbelievable and sometimes life-changing return on your otherwise small investment.

One such example is a journey that occurred over ten years ago…

Liz: I remember a trip to North Island in the Seychelles. We stayed in a small bungalow, and our house manager was a young man from Zimbabwe, Clever Zulu.

He made me feel like a princess. He did so much for us and made the best cappuccinos! In the morning, at a prearranged time, Clever would arrive, ring a bell, quietly enter, begin his preparation of our breakfast, and ask us what we would like to do for the day. Since, for me, knowing and understanding people is like food, air, and water, cappuccino was simply not enough. I wanted more. I asked him about his background, his family, and his dreams. I suggested that the next morning he arrive in his running clothes so we could run together. And he did.

We ran through this beautiful island, discussing books. He was reading the autobiographies of both Benjamin Franklin and Thomas Jefferson, literature that I would not typically read due to its dense nature. We also discussed life and explored philosophies and principles that lead to success. At that time, it just so happened that I was working with Deepak Chopra, Bob Proctor, Mark Victor Hansen, Cynthia Kersey, and some of the greatest motivational success coaches in the world. I was filming a show and writing a curriculum called "The Power to Have It All." My time with

Clever touched me deeply as I ventured into his world and listened to his stories and dreams. I was inspired to give to this hungry, optimistic soul.

RADICAL *thought*

"Giving connects two people, the giver and the receiver, and this connection gives birth to a new sense of belonging." – Deepak Chopra

Upon my return home, I gathered up the reams of success literature that I had – tapes, CDs, videos in a box filled to the brim and headed for the Seychelles. I saw it as the beginnings of a success library to give those working on the island access to literature to support their dreams. Ten years later, on a flight back from NYC after countless business meetings, I was feeling a bit down, alone, and suffering from fatigue. I read through my emails during the flight and chose to read a few that I would typically delete or pass over, as they were not mission critical; rather they were inspirational emails that arrived with regularity. Then I saw one from Clever, my Seychelles jogging partner. I opened it up and read the uplifting passage enclosed.

I decided to visit the site I was directed to, Absolute Abundance, by Clever Zulu. I was astonished by what I found. Books he had written, PowerPoint presentations he'd assembled, success principles for the hospitality industry, and so much more. I watched his video clips and began to cry. I figured in that moment, if he can do it in Zimbabwe and maintain optimism, drive, and the determination to overcome, so could I!

I sent him an email letting him know how often I think of him and how I had just gone to his site and saw all that he had created. I also told him how proud I was of him and how much I had needed to see his video and be reminded of what I already know. Within minutes, I received his response. He said, "Liz, don't you remember, you were my inspiration? You sent me all of those wonderful books and programs years ago, and believed in me and my dream." A tidal wave of emotion came over me as I saw how the simplest act of giving had touched another's life so dramatically and in return lifted my spirits in a time when I needed to be reminded of what is possible. So who really received the gift? I guess we both did. But right now, I kind of think I got the motherload.

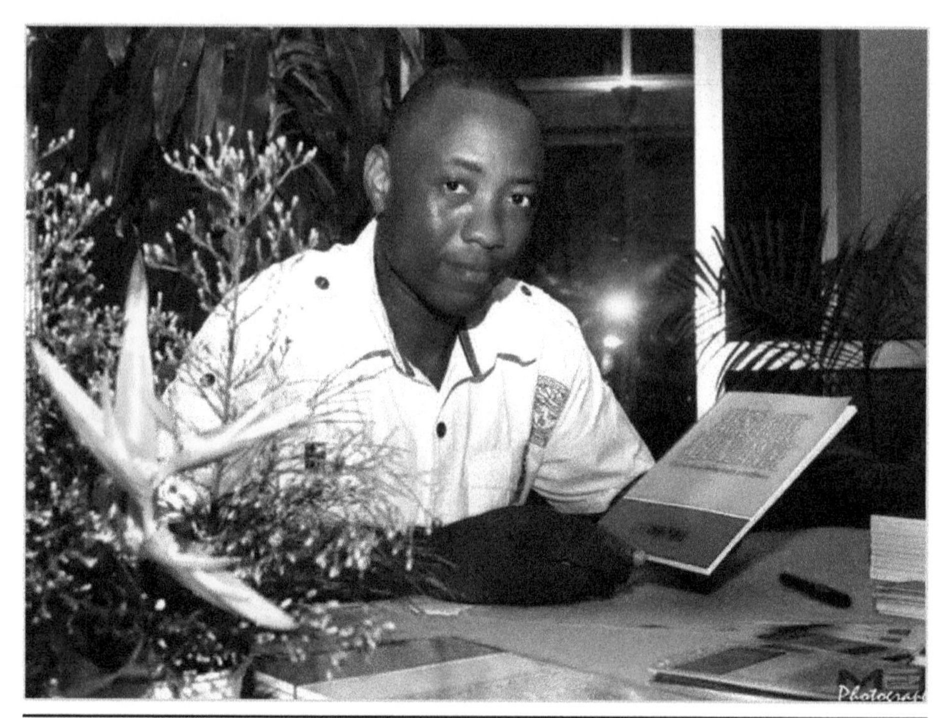

Author Clever Zulu, www.absoluteabundantia.com

It's the little things and the big things; it's all the opportunities we take advantage of to give back to one another. It is an incredible way to build a net worth of moments and memories that give back to you when you least expect it.

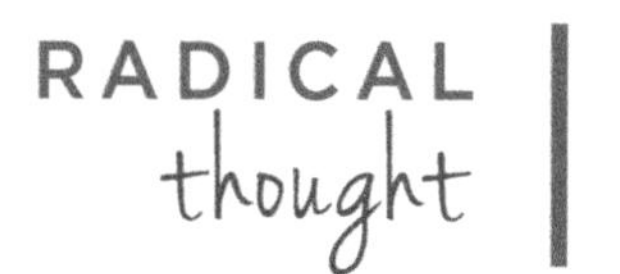

Radical giving is giving in hopes of changing the life of another. It is selfless, it is in the moment, and it is magnetic because it attracts something magnificent in return.

Whether it is through our skincare line, which helps women feel beautiful, or through this book, which will help people live beautifully, we all have a duty and a higher calling to be the difference and flex our giving muscles. Mahatma Gandhi summarizes our pillars for living a radical life when he says, "It's the action, not the fruit of the action, that's important. You have to do the right thing. It may not be in your power; it may not be in your time, that there'll be any fruit. But that doesn't mean you stop doing the right thing. You may never know what results come from your action. But if you do nothing, there will be no result."

Only when you welcome in a high willingness to say yes and act accordingly can you truly become a radical success story. It begins with little things that add up to huge things that eventually make the difference in the lives of us all.

Say the Radical Yes to giving because you can.

Say the Radical Yes to giving and watch your world transform.

Radical Recap:

To work towards Radical Giving, always remember that:

1. Radical Giving is a game of inches. You can be a great difference maker by giving in small portions. It doesn't take a home-run swing to leave a mark on humanity.

2. Become a soldier in search of opportunities to give. Then recruit other soldiers to make a similar difference in the lives of others.

3. The occasions to give are endless. Look around you. Open a door, give an unexpected compliment, or offer a warm smile to a stranger. It is the little things in life that can make the biggest difference.

4. A wonderful byproduct of giving is that you and your health benefit.

5. It is in giving that we receive. So give and feel the abundance light up inside of you.

Chapter 17: RADICAL ABUNDANCE

We reach for it wholeheartedly, and at the same time can doubt that it is there.

It is our friend that plays hide-and-seek and requires our constant attention to take the form that we desire.

It is powerful enough to drive careers, love, family, and giving at levels that can move our world.

It is the golden ring that changes shape and form depending on the age and stage of our life.

It carries its own unique frequency and station, beckoning for us to tune in to welcome its presence.

It is a double-edged sword of darkness and sorrow if it is abused and not used to create more of its kind for all whom we touch.

Have you tuned in to your channel of abundance?

Throughout our journey, we learn more everyday about how to give, how to love, and how to use our radical abundance to create more for those around us. That is a calling card for the entire Radical army. Radical is a state of mind. It is the way someone gracefully walks through the world, and because they have been here, the world is a better place. As you apply a radical prescription to your own life, the ingredients come together to position you to become a soldier, a torch barer of sorts that illuminates the flames of others, and eventually lights the world on fire. The end game is abundance. We will feel complete once we obtain an abundance of love, of security, of friendship and health. So recognizing that abundance is the destination, these final few chapters will help to give you the ingredients to get there.

We exude radical. We are radical. And so are you. You just need to say YES to the person that you truly are and want to be, and shy away from the doubts that cloud your vision. It is time for you to embrace the radical within you. It is time you mix these ingredients together in a specific and prescriptive manner to cure the ailing world. We need healing. It is time to replace war with peace, sorrow with love, depression with happiness, frowns with the brightest of smiles.

Remember: You can. You will. You are a radical human being.

To this point, we shared the ingredients that have created a radical life for us. The formula is here. The pages leading to this chapter offer a carefully constructed recipe with handpicked ingredients to secure your radicalness. You may feel as if you need different portions of each ingredient. Some of us lack love in our life, others passion. Some of us do not say "yes" enough, while others feel like they are missing on the opportunity to give to others. Whatever the case may be, recognizing your potential and also your needs is essential to your growth.

So welcome radical abundance into your life... there is truly no time like the present.

Abundance. Most dictionaries will tell you that it often refers to "a large quantity of something." Abundance is not just in reference to money, but in building a large quantity of the love you want, the health for which you strive, the balance you need, the friendships you desire, the love for which you search, the mentors you require to grow, and the job you covet. It could literally be anything. But it cannot be everything. In fact, abundance in and of itself requires harmony. We each maintain a responsibility to be wise in our choice of where we find abundance.

Think of it this way. Too many friends leave little time for the ones that truly matter. Too much money disconnects you from the rest of the world. Too much work pulls you away from those you love. Abundance without synchronicity creates a void.

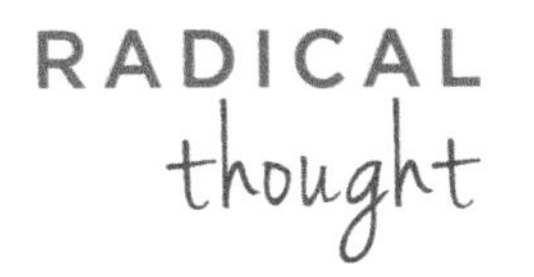

Abundance is like an anchor: if properly weighted, it can keep you in place. If over weighted, it can drag you to the bottom of the ocean.

First we want to say that wanting more is not a bad thing. Rather it is the opposite. In this capacity, we have been raised with faulty beliefs. Wanting more is your soul's calling to express itself in a greater way. It's spirit. Your spiritual DNA, which is the passionate fabric of your being, is perfect, and that perfection within you is often seeking expression through you. It strives to express itself in a greater way. You want to grow. You don't want to grow just to get. You want to grow to express yourself in a greater way. So it's great to feel happy with what you've got, but never completely satisfied if you feel there is more within you that wants to be expressed through you. Never being fully satisfied with the results we obtain is a function of believing that we have more to give. We want to get better results.

When we were little kids our grandma said, "You should be satisfied with what you've got." Well, we've come to find that our wonderful grandma was mistaken. Dissatisfaction gave us the incandescent light. Dissatisfaction gave us the ability to build a life that we love. Dissatisfaction gave us the drive to share Radical with you because it burned within us as something we had to express.

We were not satisfied with Radical Skincare sitting on our bathroom counter for only ourselves, our mom, and our friends to enjoy the benefits. So we launched it in retail around the world. We still weren't satisfied because we knew that Radical could reach more people deeply and transform their lives if they knew what was behind it and us. So we took Radical Skincare to television so we could reach more people and tell the story, which we do on QVC.

But still we were not satisfied. We knew that through QVC we could share the science that can change your skin, but there was not enough time on QVC to share the science to change your life. So we created a Radical Access club that people can join to transform not only their skin, but also their life. There we have the ability to share proprietary wellness solutions that we don't take to retail or to television. We have the ability to engage in a conversation to coach and empower people to have a life they love. Radical Access for those who want more and want to be involved with us can become a part of the mission that changes people's skin and life. You can be our partner and experience life-changing abundance born out of a desire to do and be more, because together we can.

Think about the art of invention. It is often bred from dissatisfaction. Inventors did not create solutions because they were unhappy; they were simply dissatisfied with the results they received. Edison gave us incandescent light since he obviously wasn't satisfied with the kerosene lamp or a wax candle. He illuminated the whole darn world. The Wright Brothers weren't satisfied with the horse and buggy. They wanted to fly.

The goal post of abundance is constantly moving because we're constantly changing and evolving. Look back on your life to date and think of your abundance. Each moment that is loved and cherished is a lustrous pearl. String the pearls together and you create a beautiful necklace. Symbolically you will see before you a life well lived.

It's truly the stringing together of moment after moment after moment. The luster of that necklace can only be judged by what you are personally passionate about and what is meaningful to you. It could be travel. It could be children. It could be touching people. It could be money. It could be helping people. It could be hobbies. It could be homes or art. It could be ultimate fitness. It could be giving. It could be any number of things. But through your pearls, your necklace, your life radiates and shines with unbelievable amounts of abundance, coming in all different shapes and sizes.

Celebrated author and speaker Dr. Wayne Dyer said, "Abundance is not something we acquire. It is something we tune into." We can do that in a number of different ways. But it often starts with using your senses like listening and looking around you to see where the abundance may be. Abundance is truly everywhere. It surrounds us and engulfs our lives. But we often look past it, even when it is staring us right in the eyes. Once you tune in, you will find yourself primed to manifest a life filled with radical abundance. And ultimately that is our goal with this book. Through our journey, we have determined there are very specific and enormously powerful ways to tune in and attract abundance. It is our hope that if you decide to tune in to these four radical channels, you'll begin to vibrate at a different frequency, at a radical frequency.

Having learned so much from the great Bob Proctor, and interviewing him specifically for this chapter, we felt it only appropriate to share his insightful and meaningful words on each of these action-oriented steps.

The four keys to obtaining radical abundance are:

1. **Goal Setting:** *Set a goal that is big enough to both scare you and excite you.*

2. **The Law of Attraction:** *Be clear and control that which you focus on.*

3. **Visualization:** *Create an emotionally engaging and blockbuster movie of your dreams in your mind.*

4. **Consistency in Your Behavior:** *Practice and implement these skills daily.*

These strategies collide at the intersection of *radical* and *abundance* to harness an energy that supports the creation of the life you want to live. Once you are practicing a life filled with passion and purpose, these are the steps that infuse your life with strength, meaning, happiness, success, and unparalleled abundance. We invite you to become a radical thinker and believer, and it starts with setting goals, increasing your vibration, attracting abundance, visualizing your dreams, and being consistent in your behavior.

Radical Recap:

To achieve Radical Abundance, always remember that:

1. It is important for you to believe that you deserve all that you desire.
2. Abundance changes depending on the position of your life. Define what it looks like for you now, so that you can see the opportunities to embrace in front of you.
3. Your abundance is a benefit to all whom you touch. The more you have, the more you have to share.

"You are worthy of a life
even greater than
you can imagine.
Dare to dream it.
Dare to live it."
–Rick Tamlyn

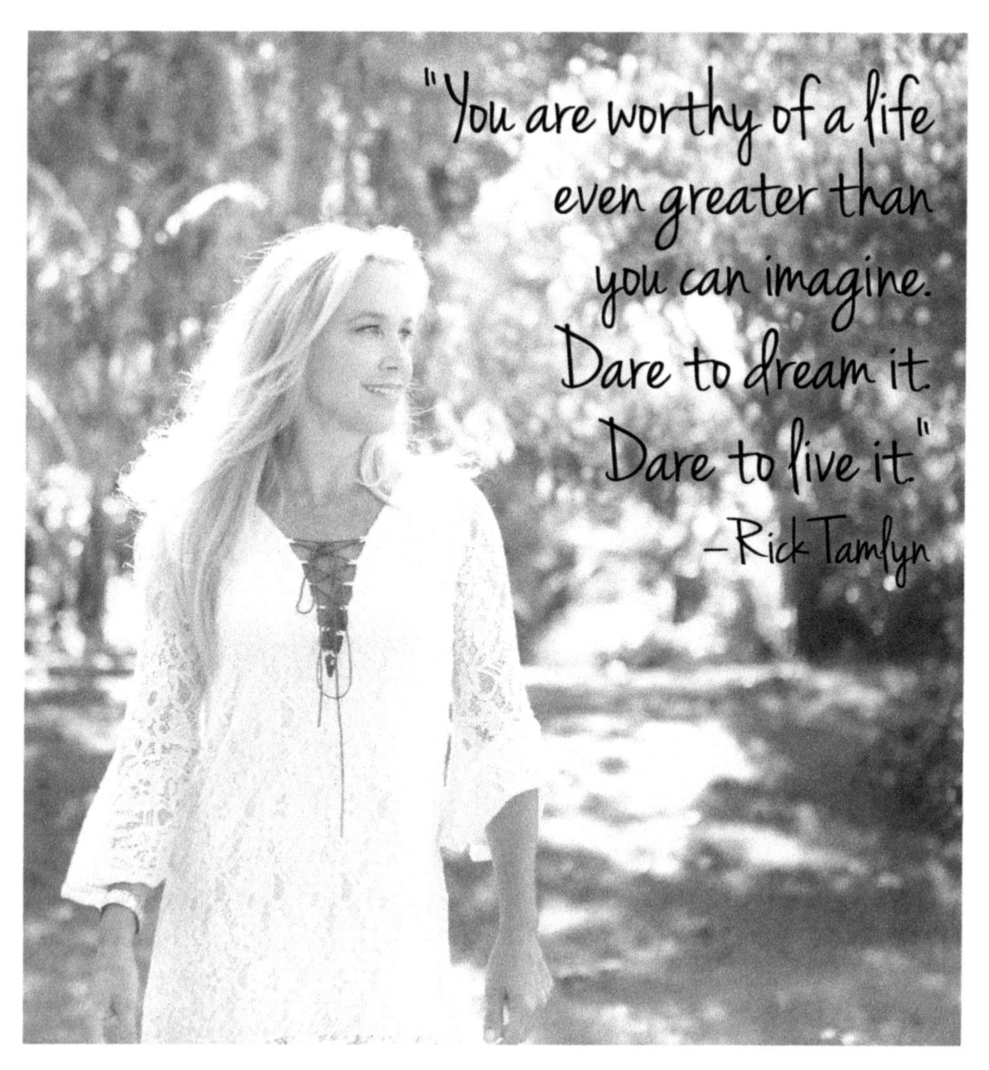

Chapter 18:
RADICAL GOAL SETTING

Abundance begins with setting goals. Goals are those special and defined targets for which we aim. They are everywhere and can be anything. To reach a state of abundance, you have to first decide what that looks like.

How many times have you set a goal, only to find yourself fall short or allow it to fizzle out, like a dimly burning candle? It happens far too often. But while we often fall short of our goals, we rarely take the time to evaluate and assess exactly why those goals are close but remain unreached. The goal you set should scare you and excite you at the same time. Don't take that sentence lightly. Too often we set goals that we know we can achieve and that truly do not inspire us or change our lives. If you are going to dream, then dream big. Now. Because if you don't, you may end up looking back at the you that you *could* have become. What do you have to lose?

To this point, we assume we are on the same page and have agreed to say *yes* to setting goals that are inspirational and life changing; goals that give you the passion and purpose to make it through the storms you may encounter, and the will to do it and focus.

Focus is like a lantern, guiding us through the journey to abundance and creating a burning light that attracts others to join our journey. As we set goals, the key is to focus not just on the overarching goal, but also the segments or notches of that goal. We believe in the power of chunking down big goals into more manageable and bite size pieces. Look at the big picture as just a series of small pictures. Break your goal down into smaller and more achievable goals. And then focus on your growth and those smaller goals on a daily basis. This will help keep your focus and your goals at the forefront of your mind.

Let's assume your goal is to find love. While that may seem like a lofty goal, it is one tantamount to human nature. But you wouldn't wake up one day, leave your house, and aimlessly wander the streets looking, right? Of course not. You'd likely chunk it down by telling your friends and colleagues you'd love to be set up. You might inform those around you that you are ready to welcome in a life partner. Or maybe you'd join a dating website, or social media, or some other medium. You would meet some candidates; you'd go on a first date, and hopefully a second one. Phone calls, emails, and long evenings would ensue for you and your new interest. Eventually, as trust, familiarity, and respect grew, you'd likely feel as if you were in love. But it started with baby steps and manageable little pieces that grew into something much larger. Pieces like creating a vision board of what is indicative of the qualities you want in a man; pieces like writing down a description of your new love, what he or she does, what his or her primary characteristics and values are; pieces like writing the script of the movie of your future love that you would like to see with the intention of being clear to the universe that this is the wish list that you would like delivered. Join a few activity groups with other like-minded people and put yourself out there and tell friends you would love to meet someone.

Goal setting is often supported by the fact that it creates ownership of an idea or a dream. It is not just fantasizing; it is reality. Scientists often refer to this concept of ownership as the endowment effect, which is the common practice of ascribing more value to things just because we own them. This occurs when we take ownership of something and it becomes part of our sense of identity.

Cornell University researchers demonstrated the power of the endowment effect in a study where they first gave each person in a controlled group a coffee mug. They then asked if each person would like to trade his or her coffee mug for a piece of chocolate. Almost all of the participants turned down this offer, choosing to keep the mug. The researchers then reversed the trial, first giving a controlled group chocolate and then offering to trade it for the coffee mugs. Once again, almost the entire group declined the trade. In this study, researchers found the endowment effect in full force. It was never about the preferred object, but rather about keeping what they already had.

Bob Proctor shares with us: "Goals are what you want. Most people set goals to get what they think they can do or what they think they need. When setting a goal, follow the quiet voice within and go by the feelings that are coming to you that excite you and would be a game changer in your life. Once you set the goal in your consciousness and you have a plan, know that the plan rarely takes you there in just the way that you thought. You have to continually change the plan and evolve. *You change the plan, but you don't change the goal. Because the goal needs to be at the core of your heart's desire.*"

Bob says, "You've got to go after what you want. When you go after what you want, you've got to realize that your memory's not going to take you there. You've got to realize that wants start out with fantasies. You've got to fantasize. So you build the picture in your mind of this beautiful place that you're going to go to, this beautiful thing that you're going to do. All great goals start out with fantasies. The Wright Brothers fantasized. Edison fantasized. Sir Edmund Hillary fantasized. They built a fantasy in their mind. They were even reluctant to tell anybody because they knew everybody would think they were crazy. When that happens, you know you're on the right track."

When we fantasize, when we set and then see our goal, we may want to keep it to ourselves for a while. Like jewels in our jewel box, we bring them out only when we feel that the person we are sharing them with can appreciate them. Goals are sacred. Treat them that way, and don't let others toss them around on the waves of disbelief and cynicism. Hold that beautiful vision as close as you would a newborn. Your goals need your protection, they need you to feed them and nurture them and help them grow to their ultimate potential. Then they will manifest and shine, a splendor for you and others to enjoy.

TURN YOUR FANTASY INTO A THEORY ON ITS WAY TO BECOMING A GOAL

Initially, your goal should be born in fantasy. When you turn it into an actionable plan with descriptors it gives it a life of its own. Once you convert the imaginable to the real, you actually give dreams teeth, which then turn them into a goal. You have to ask yourself two important questions:

Am I able to do this?

4. Am I willing to do this?

"All things are possible. All science and all theology tell you that you are infinite; you have infinite potential. You are able. Then you have to go to the second test: am I willing to do what is required? Your best sometimes isn't good enough. You've got to do what's required. When you decide to do that which is required, you pass the acid test and the theory turns into a goal and you turn that over to the universal mind," says our friend Bob.

Bob continues: "William James, from Harvard, said, 'Implant it in the garden of your subconscious mind.' When it's planted in the garden of the subconscious mind, the laws of the universe go to work. When you really understand that, that's when you start to move in the right direction."

RADICAL thought

Andrew Carnegie, the wealthiest man in the world in 1908, said, "Any idea that is held in the mind, that's emphasized, that's either feared or revered, will begin at once to clothe itself in the most convenient and appropriate form available."

Consider the example of Peter O'Toole, who played in the movie *Lawrence of Arabia*. He did such a phenomenal job he was nominated for an Academy Award. Listen to what Lawrence said about dreams. He said, 'All men dream, but not equally. Those who dream by night, in the dusty recesses of their mind, waken in the day to find that it was vanity. But the dreamers of the day are dangerous individuals, for they may act their dreams with open eyes to make it possible. This I did.'"

When asked what we can do to become radical goal setters, Bob reminded us: "You have to be very quiet and listen to what's going on inside. Sometimes it takes a while. You might have to take a half-hour to an hour every day. The best time is early in the morning. Go sit by yourself in a quiet place and say, 'What do I really want to do? What would I love doing?' It starts out as a fantasy. Everything inside of you tells you this is crazy, it'll never happen. That's when you've got to look at radical individuals of the past and realize that they had the same little mental hurdle to overcome.

They decided that they would make it happen when it was nothing but a mere fantasy.

"And so they just put it in writing. They wrote it out in a clear, concise statement so that if somebody else read it, they would get the same picture as the dreamer, as the one with the fantasy. Then they had to turn it into a theory. They started to think about it seriously and they started moving ahead. They laid out a plan knowing the plan probably isn't going to take them there but it is a starting point.

"There is beauty in writing it down. Writing causes thinking. You're creating an image of it. Those images are planted in the cells in your brain. Those cells increase in amplitude of vibration and the picture of your goal splashes all over the screen of your mind. The trick is to keep that picture on the screen of your mind as often as possible, because when you do, that's when you're giving energy to it. Energy is flowing to and through you. It never stops. When you're thinking of your goal, the energy that's flowing through you is moving toward your goal."

RADICAL *thought*

Emerson said, "The only thing that can grow is the thing you give energy to."

"You couldn't share your idea if you didn't have it," Bob says. "It's not that you're going to get it – you've got it and you've got to think like you've got it. Then you must turn that over to your heart, to the heart of hearts, to the emotional side of your personality. You let yourself get emotionally involved in the idea. When you've got it in your heart, then you are on the way. You are in that vibration. You are on the frequency of the good that you desire and you can share it."

Researchers Ad Kleingeld and Heleen Van Mierlo conducted a large analysis over the course of thirty-eight studies on goal setting. They found there is a pattern between goals that work and those that don't. In an article titled "The Science of Goal Setting," Vanessa Van Edwards interprets the results to find that goals that are reached are often:

1. **Measureable:** They should have a clear beginning and ending and remain quantifiable. *Radical clarity:* Be specific with dates and times.

2. **Actionable:** You should understand your wants and recognize the journey to achieve them. *Radical knowledge:* Am I willing and am I able?

3. **Realistic:** They should be achievable and aligned with your life.[21] *Radical inspiration:* Tap into your heart's desire and consider that which lights you up with passion and purpose, but also that which scares and excites you at the same time.

Goals will always come in many different shapes and sizes. They are rarely a one-size-fits-all proposition. You'll always find yourself ahead of the game if you have set goals. Remember, abundance begins with radical goal setting. Fail to plan and you plan to fail. Writing your goals and seeing what is necessary to achieve them is important. Fuel the fire, allowing it to gain momentum and burn brightly. Once we burn at a high temperature, we create the energy that radiates within. Only then can we welcome in the next piece to manifesting radical abundance – the law of attraction. But first we must set our goals to create what we really want.

SETTING YOUR GOAL: WHAT DO YOU REALLY WANT?

The purpose of goals is not to get but to grow. The energy of abundance constantly moves through you. Owning a goal as a picture in your mind is one of the *most* important things that we will share with you in this book. Goals are misunderstood and tend to carry with them a weighty and lackluster hue. Since childhood, goals are often "given" to us and imposed upon us. Typically, they were not born of our heart's desire, but from the "shoulds" and "have to's," which are not so sexy or exciting.

So it is important to put that aside for a moment and erase the chalkboard of your mind as it relates to goals, creating space for what is absolutely essential to your achievements.

First, you need to know what you want.

There are three types of goals that can be illustrated through the visual of a three-story house:

1. **Basement Goals:** These consist of those goals you think you can achieve. You have accomplished them already and just want them to be a bit better. But they hold no real creativity, inspiration, or love.

2. **Second Floor Goals:** You can see what is possible given what you know today, and you stretch yourself a bit but still play it safe. It is within the realm of what you know.

3. **Roof Deck Goals:** These are the meaningful ones. They carry no ceiling and give wings to your heart's desire. Your dream, fantasy, and vision of what you really want can live and breathe here. Your goal is big and you have no idea how you will get there, and it may even feel a little bit crazy. But the vision of it is exciting, creates passion, and you can see yourself with it.

Your goal must reside in the present tense. It is the "I am so happy and grateful NOW that..."

And it must have a date attached so that you have informed the universe of a timetable that works for you.

For example, it could sound like: "I am so happy and grateful NOW that I am passionately in love and alive with my husband/partner surrounded by friends and family. I am inspired daily by my business and am empowering millions of people worldwide with our products, services, and message by June 2016. I am feeling healthy and great at 128 lbs. and am having so much fun on a daily basis. Our billion-dollar company drops a 25 percent net profit, which allows us to give more and change more lives worldwide by 2018. I have x$ in my account and a home that I visit in x, y, or z. I travel and experience different cultures and that fills my heart with joy..."

Break this goal down by writing it on a card that you keep in your wallet, purse, or on your mirror, helping to constantly trigger this image.

What image? Every word on this card will correspond to a picture or a descriptive page of what your goal looks and feels like to you. Take this exercise very seriously, because you will create what you write down if you work to constantly remind yourself of those goals that you set.

So for example: "Passionately in love and alive with my husband..."

Create a separate sheet and write down exactly what you want in a husband or relationship, what you do, where you go, what you like together, your interests, his dominant traits, etc. Have fun with it and write your goals on this page.

The same will be true for your family, business, and anything and everything that you choose to write by hand on paper. That's right. By hand – the old-fashioned way. Writing causes thinking and reflection and engages many of your senses at one time, which makes it a powerful tool to manifest. As you do this, your mind will act as a switching station and reignite the omni-colored dream in your heart.

You might like to travel and enjoy different cultures. So on a separate paper you might create a list of the places that you'd envision traveling to and what those experiences would feel like. The word travel will then light up all of the pictures in your mind of where you want to go and what those experiences will look like.

This little exercise is the most important secret to creating a life that you love. Success is directly related to speaking, seeing, and living exactly what you want.

After this exercise, put your goal card everywhere. Read it morning and night. Put it in your wallet so that every time you open it you trigger that goal. Put it in the medicine cabinet, use it as a screen saver, save it in your closet. Put it in as many places as possible and give it the needed energy to exist because anything that we give energy to will take form.

I was in the Bahamas with my friend Ana. She told me story after story about her upbringing in Venezuela and how her grandmother overcame seemingly impossible odds to bring her to where she is today. Her grandmother used to always say to her: "Speak only of what you want and say only the positive. You never know when the angels are listening and will say 'Amen!'"

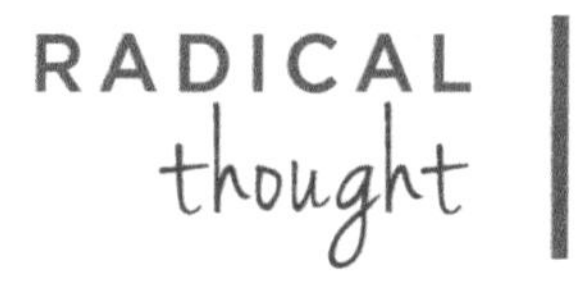

Speak only of what you want and say only the positive. You never know when the angels are listening and will say "Amen!"

Over our Radical journey there have been countless stories and emails from people who have followed these powerful but simple steps and watched miracles occur. What most people don't understand is that these are not miracles, but rather the universe's response to our clear desire and attention to the goals we set.

Radical Recap:

To reach your full capacity to set Radical Goals, always remember that:

1. Take time to think, to imagine, and to fantasize about what you really want.
2. Decide if you are willing and able to do what it takes to get there.
3. Write your goals in the present tense and be specific with dates and amounts.
4. Set goals that are big enough to scare and excite you so that you have the emotional passion and purpose behind you to fuel their creation.
5. Put your goal card everywhere to re-trigger the image in your mind.
6. Remember: you can change the plan, but you don't change the goal. Because the goal needs to be at the core of your heart's desire."

Chapter 19: RADICAL ATTRACTION

Albert Einstein said, "Everything is energy and that's all there is to it. Match the frequency of the reality you want and you cannot help but get that reality. It can be no other way. This is not philosophy. This is physics."

The second pathway to radical abundance is through the law of attraction. In one form or another, most of us are familiar with the law of attraction. It is a simple yet potent way to welcome in our goals and lead us towards abundance. Any meaningful prescription to create a radical life includes a magnetizing behavior to attract all that you want into your life.

Author Stephen Richards said, "When you concentrate your energy purposely on the future possibility that you aspire to realize, your energy is passed on to it and it is attracted to you with a force stronger than the one you directed towards it." In each of us lies an abundance of energy. That energy can be given to any number of opportunities within our life.

With that said, radical abundance calls for each of us to focus on what we desire. We have all heard of the law of attraction. In its simplest form, think of how many times you've thought of a person and then heard from him or her. Or on how many occasions you thought you were going to fall, and found yourself on the ground just a few minutes later? There are many examples we can point to in our everyday life that represent the power of this law. In life, there are very few coincidences. The world brings us together in a purposeful and meaningful way. At some level, we attract that which we want, but in reality we attract that which we focus on.

YOU ARE WHAT YOU SAY YOU ARE, AND YOU WILL CREATE WHAT YOU BELIEVE

Your power resides within your mind, and harnessing that power in a controlled manner will drive you in the direction of abundance.

It is absolutely clear to us that you can attract your abundant life with the correct mindset. The law of attraction is not just a choice, but rather it is your choice to make. Your journey begins when you wholeheartedly decide to focus on and vibrate at a level that welcomes your desired goals and your success. Once you are an adult, everything in life is a choice. Our thoughts are the one thing over which we have absolute control. The law of attraction allows you to attract whatever it is you're thinking about. No matter your situation, your challenges, your perceived limitations, or even the current backdrop of your life, the law of attraction supports your ability to control your mind. And it is through the energy vibrating within your mind that you can manifest and welcome abundance.

But more important than the law of attraction is the law of vibration.

Bob Proctor offers us a unique view of the law of attraction. He says, "What most people don't understand is that the law of attraction is a secondary law. The primary law is the law of vibration. Your mind and body vibrate. It's a mass of molecules operating under a very high speed of vibration. The ideas that you hold in your mind and turn over to your subconscious mind dictate the vibration you're in. Feeling is a word we invented to describe our awareness of the vibration we're in. If you do not feel good, it's because you're in a bad vibration. You are entertaining a negative thought. When you feel good, you're in a good vibration and you're entertaining a good thought.

"Now, understand [that] the vibration you're in is going to dictate what you attract. You can only attract the energy with which you're in harmony. If you're in a bad vibration, you'll never attract good energy. You'll attract bad energy. If you're in a bad vibration and you're complaining and finding everything that is wrong, you're going to attract people with similar behavior. You'll have a lot in common. And because you have a lot in common, you talk about it. But the same is true when you entertain positive ideas. You will attract positive people. People will come into your life that you would have never met otherwise, and they will be there to help you. It's like there's a network of positive people helping positive people all over the world, which you and I are connected to."

At what frequency do you vibrate?

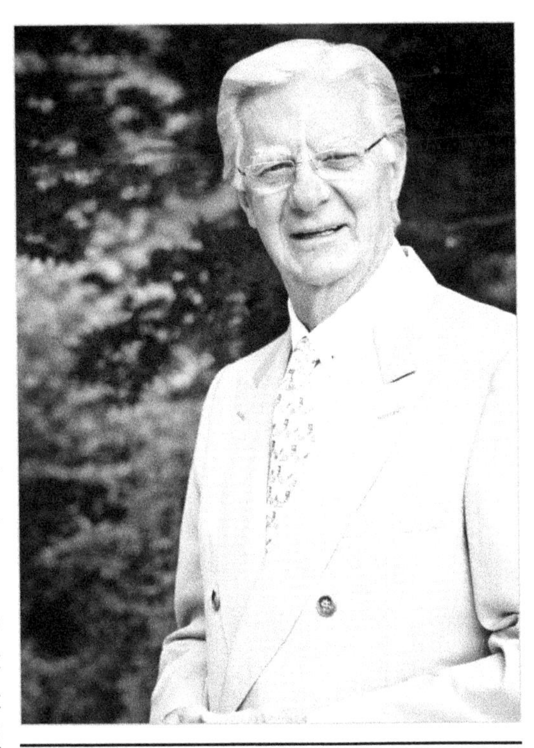

Bob Proctor

This remains an important question to consider. We all have the ability to turn the dial and tune in to the frequency of abundance. There are times when we don't vibrate at a positive frequency. During those times, we bury the law of attraction in our negative mindsets. But with positive thoughts and a focused mind, we can tune in to a better frequency, one that is aligned with what we choose to attract.

The law of attraction is a gift to each of us. But it is only a gift when we give it the energy that we can truly understand, and then elevate its fundamental power to welcome in radical abundance. It is our choice. So, wake up every day and choose to vibrate at a positive frequency, one supported by constructive and encouraging energy that opens the doors for what you radically desire.

If the first step is to write down your goals, the second step is to make the very important decision to vibrate at a frequency that attracts the stepping-stones to focus on what you want to do. As these opportunities coincide with one another, we begin to elevate our opportunity to obtain radical abundance.

Radical Recap:

To engage the law of attraction, always remember to:

1. Read positive and affirming passages.
2. Meditate and shift your focus to what you want.
3. Surround yourself with positive people that vibrate at positive frequencies.
4. Laugh. Often.
5. Control your thoughts: dismiss those that do not support what you want and redirect your energy towards those that do.
6. Be mindful and conscious of the real estate in your mind that you give to your thoughts.

"Life is not measured by the breaths you take,
but by the moments that take
your breath away."
–Maya Angelou

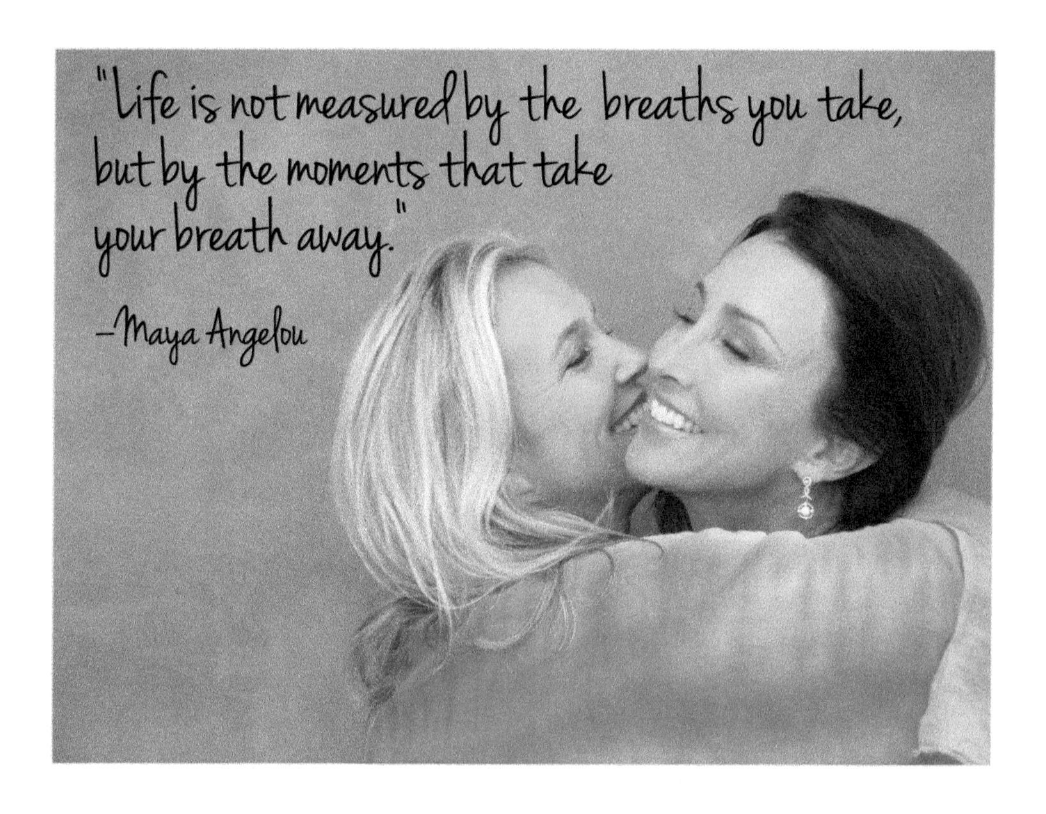

Chapter 20: RADICAL INTENTION

Author Robert Collier said, "Visualize this thing that you want, see it, feel it, believe in it. Make your mental blueprint, and begin to build."

Goal setting and the law of attraction will propel you on the path to radical abundance. Start by writing your dreams and wants down (goal setting) and then vibrating at a frequency that attracts your goals (The Law of Attraction). Then see them (visualization) and be present with them (consistency) to allow them to manifest into a fulfilling life that often exceeds your highest hopes and aspirations (abundance).

The equation is pretty simple:

Abundance =

Goal Setting + Law of Attraction + Visualization + Consistency

Goal setting and attraction are the planning part of your journey. Figuring out your destination and then focusing on attracting it are what will help to place you in a position to visualize your goals.

Visualization requires planning. If you don't know where you are today, it is difficult to know how to get where you want to be tomorrow. That essential comparison will not only define the gap, but also begin the process of bridging it. If you are unaware of the size of the gap, you'll never truly know how far you need to travel to get around it.

Before you can even begin visualizing where you strive to reach, essential consideration should be given to assessing exactly where you'd like to dock your ship at the end of the long voyage. If you do not truly understand your endgame, or where you want to anchor your life, you'll find yourself traveling the open seas with little direction. Undirected visualization is almost as detrimental as no visualization at all. So before we can truly tune in and welcome the images of our future, it is essential to devote time to self-reflection, evaluation, and assessment. The most important questions you can ask yourself are:

- *Where are you?*
- *Where do you want to go?*
- *What are you doing?*
- *What is working?*
- *What is not working?*

These simple questions and answers can radically transform your life. The answers to these questions will help you pinpoint exactly where you are on the map. You'll then be primed to begin the visualization process.

WHERE ARE YOU? WHERE DO YOU WANT TO GO?

One day we were very frustrated with our Radical Skincare journey. Prestige skincare was a much bigger beast than we had ever imagined with a longer timeframe than we envisioned. With our arms thrown up in the air in utter disdain, we spoke to Bob about where we were and how long it would take to get exactly where we wanted to be. We had a feeling that we were not exactly on schedule. Then he said something to us that put it all in perspective.

He told us that we first needed to get really honest with ourselves, take a look at where we were, and decide where we wanted to go. He said, "If you were in NYC and your goal was to be in Los Angeles, and you found yourself in Nevada on your way there, would you be all up in arms because you were in Nevada but on your way? Of course not! You would know that you were on your journey, with your end goal clearly planted in the GPS of your mind."

You never know if there will be detours that cause delays, road closures, storms, or other unforeseen circumstances. What matters is that the end goal, the picture, and the dream in your mind remain, and that you put one foot in front of the other and advance. You never know how close you are to the finish line until you take that last step. Winners never quit and quitters never win. It is the radical perseverance of a worthy ideal that embodies your passion and purpose that will take you there. So don't curse the journey and the road you are on, but instead give more energy to the image in your mind that you are in pursuit of, and breathe life into the dream that awaits you.

WHAT ARE YOU DOING? WHAT IS WORKING? WHAT IS NOT WORKING?

The definition of insanity is doing the same thing over and over and expecting a different result. Look at your life. You are the expert. What habits, people, thoughts, and choices support you and which ones don't? You have the luxury of looking at these ingredients and choosing to be aware and limit those that are not supporting your journey. It is not a pleasant exercise at times, and may require us to muster up a bit of radical courage and face the terror barrier. Remember Joseph Campbell's admonition: "The cave that I fear to enter holds the treasure I seek."

RADICAL *thought* | Take an inventory of the results in your life and start doing more of what is working and stop doing what isn't.

It sounds simple, but too many times we proceed on automatic, doing what we think should be done even though it is proving ineffective. The other day we walked into a meeting with our consultants and said, "What are we doing? What is working and what isn't working?" We asked for an analysis of all of it, and within hours we saw the roadmap for our next steps. We had frankly been in the dark and paying for the best of the best and hoping for great results. But when they weren't there, we took to asking the five critical questions.

- *Where are we?*
- *Where do we want to go?*
- *What are we doing?*
- *What is working?*
- *What is not working?*

When we did that, we changed our strategy to get results. This can be applied in your relationships, work, friendships, or any area of your life that you feel is not delivering results.

Once you have clarity and your goal is in clear view, it is time to press the accelerator and visualize. Engage the movie in your mind like your life depends on it… because it does. Living a radical life of no excuses and no regrets depends on engaging your mind's eye and seeing what you want in living color.

The beauty is that most of the above rests in our hands. We have the power to accelerate or decelerate this growth and the eventuality of this vision. How long it takes is up to us. The truth is we know in our hearts how much we are giving to this vision and how stingy we are being by withholding the necessary ingredients. Visualization is at the root of the seeds we sow and will certainly determine the abundance of the crop that we reap.

VISUALIZATION IN ACTION

Visualization is the equivalent of power. Schedule it into your days. Just like you find time for a meeting, for meals, or for a workout, find time to visualize. Locate a quiet room. Become comfortable in that room, adjusting the lights, the sounds, the aromas, and even the temperature. Close your eyes. Work to turn down the noise that often distracts you in your daily activities. Now focus. Breathe deeply, introducing the images of what you wish to achieve. Now allow those images to expand and prosper within your mind. These images may begin fuzzy and out of focus. But as you invest more energy into these images, you will find they become clear, emphasized, and concentrated. As they receive nurturing, they will expand. One image becomes two, and two become three, and before you know it, your mind will be flooded with images. These images should be moments in time. They should be visual representations of that which you want. These images will represent your radical abundance.

Do you want a better marriage? Visualize the images you feel represent the marriage of your dreams. More walks on the beach? More intimacy? Less work? More children? A different house? The options are truly endless. But whatever you so choose, you have to focus on and visualize. It is through visualization that you can begin to water the seeds of abundance. As the seeds embed themselves into your mind, your powerful mind will begin to welcome them in and manifest them into your daily life.

Science supports the notion that we stimulate the same brain regions when we are visualizing an action as when we are actually performing that same action. For example, when you visualize raising your foot, it stimulates the same part of the brain that is activated when you raise your foot. In a study conducted by Stephen J. Page, PhD, he tested thirty-two chronic stroke patients with moderate motor deficits. During his study, part of the group physically practiced a grip-strengthening exercise for four weeks, while the other part of his group only mentally practiced the same exercise, visualizing the action and the behavior. At the conclusion of the study, the results showed almost the same exact improvement between the two groups. With nothing more than visualization of the actual activity, the first group showed almost identical strength gains as the second.

This example of visualization shows how powerful the simple task of focusing on an outcome can be. Now supplement that with actually doing it and think of the possibilities.

Bob Proctor says, "Visualization is absolutely essential to success. Imagination is the tool that allows visions to arise. Relax and let yourself hold an image of the good that you desire. If you train yourself to deliberately picture yourself with your goal and carefully examine the picture, you will attract everything that is required for the manifestation of that picture, and you'll attract them by the harmonious vibration of the law of attraction. You see – everything you want is already here. You've got to get in harmony with it. You have to accept it as it is already yours."

Howard Ruby – friend, mentor, and the husband of one of our dearest friends, Yvette Mimieux – is an extremely successful businessman who is driven to make a difference. Starting at the age of five managing his lemonade stand, working as a golf caddie at age twelve, and at twenty-four with only $1000 in his pocket, he used visualization, goal setting, and desire to create an empire worth over a billion dollars.

As the CEO of Oakwood Worldwide, the world's largest corporate-housing provider, with locations in fifty states and eighty-six countries,

Howard shared his life lessons with us over lunch. We asked him what he felt were the most critical practices that have brought him the success he enjoys today.

"Visualization is one of the most important keys to success," Howard told us. "You have to be able to see a room with four blank walls and see it fully decorated in your mind. You must visualize how your product or service can be used and why people want it. You must be able to see the end that you have in mind. And then practice seeing it daily. So whatever you desire, you have to REALLY want it. The radical difference between people who get what they want is that they really desire deeply what they want. They do whatever it takes and they hold the vision in their mind every day and see it again and again.

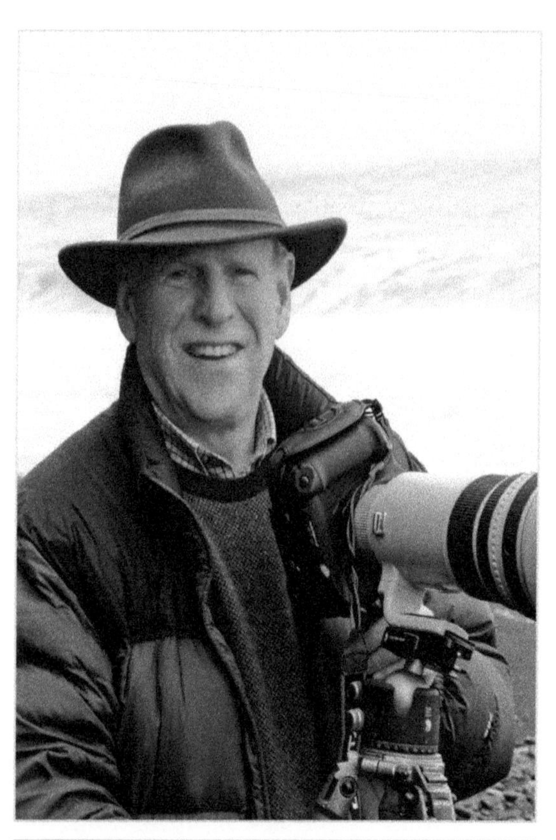

Photographer Howard Ruby in action

"A few years ago I was diagnosed with retinitis pigmentosa, a disease most people know as tunnel vision. I didn't realize I had it until I was sixty-five, and it inspired me to capture as much of our world as possible through the lens of my camera.

"Even though today my eyesight is impaired, my vision is as strong as ever. Aside from running my business, I have been taking photographs of endangered wildlife and locations around the world, in hopes of educating youth about climate change. I partnered with the National Wildlife Federation and set up Climateclassroomkids.org, with lesson plans about the changing environment around the world.

"Taking the road less traveled, going against the grain, being radical, and thinking out of the box is just the beginning. You then must have the burning

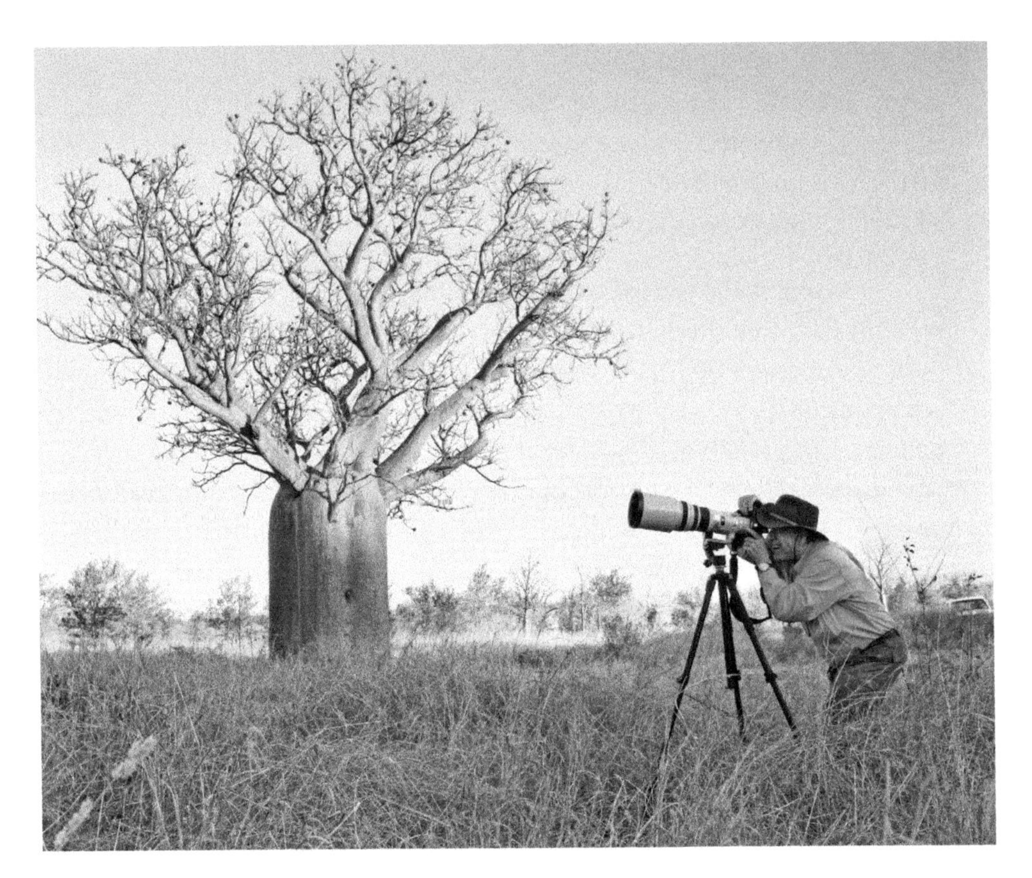

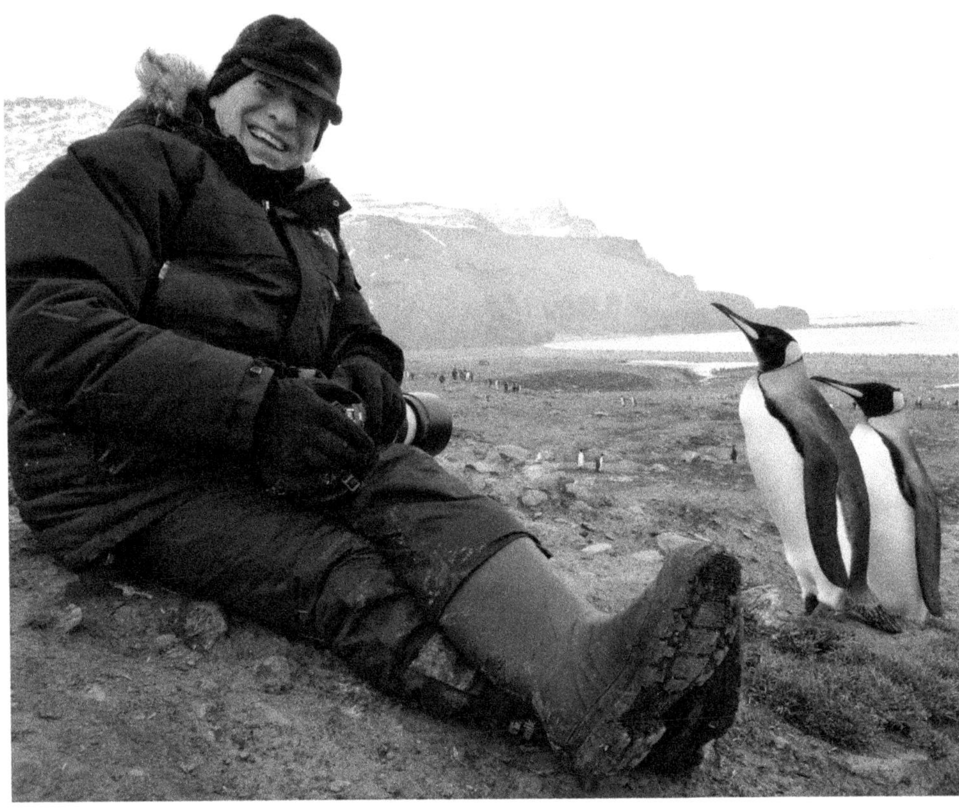

desire to create your dream, whatever that may be, and then do whatever it takes to make it happen. On your journey your greatest ally will be the vision you hold and seeing what you want in all its glory painted on the four empty walls before you."

Visualization in the face of adversity can be a challenge. On one occasion, we told Bob that we felt like we were working hard, pushing hard, and only saw incremental gain. We asked him why it took so long for us to reach our goals. He said to us, "You'll never find abundance when you are pushing against it. Force negates it. There's a law of non-resistance. What you resist persists. You don't resist anything. It's actually non-resistance. You let it happen. That's where faith comes in. If you don't have faith then you're never going to be independent and achieve abundance. You need to fearlessly and clearly hold onto your vision and surround yourself with others who are in harmony with you. So hold the image of the good that you desire and let your dream team support that vision. Visualization is the great secret to success."

Visualization is an unbelievable power within us all. And the best part is that it costs little more than our time and focus. Schedule visualization into your daily routine. Find time to sit down and dedicate your full attention to visualizing that which you so desire. Once you do so, and make it a daily habit, you'll find that what you reach for will be presented.

Radical Recap:

To better visualize your desired Radical Results, always remember to:

1. Know where you are.
2. Know where you want to go.
3. Know what is working and what is not working.
4. Do more of what is working and less of what isn't.
5. Hold onto your vision like a movie in your mind where you are the star.

Chapter 21: RADICAL CONSISTENCY

The final piece to creating a prescription for a radically abundant life is becoming consistent in your goal setting, regularly practicing the law of attraction, the law of vibration, and visualizing your ultimate dreams and success. Consistency forms habits, and it is through the formation of those habits that practices become almost subconscious norms.

Look at what you are doing daily and monthly, and determine what is working and what is not.

The goal of consistency is to form habits that support growth and evolution. When you form positive habits, you place yourself in a nutrient-rich and prosperous environment, one where you have limitless growth potential. Habits can go either way. They can support you and elevate your abundance, or they can weigh you down and suffocate your ability to develop. Habit-forming behavior is remarkably easy to create. Once an action becomes a habit, it is substantially easier to be consistent.

In the 1950s, Maxwell Maltz, a successful plastic surgeon, noticed a strange pattern among his patients. After an operation, he found that it would take the patient a minimum of twenty-one days or so to get used to his or her new face. Noticing his clients' reactions, he began to consider his own ability to adjust, change, and eventually to form a habit. In his book *Psycho-Cybernetics,* Maltz discussed his thoughts on behavioral changes by stating, "These, and many other commonly observed phenomena tend to show that it requires a minimum of about twenty-one days for an old mental image to dissolve and a new one to jell."[23] *Psycho-Cybernetics* went on to sell over 30 million copies, and Maltz's work has been quoted and referenced by almost every major self-help professional in the world.

However, Phillippa Lally, a researcher at University College London, decided to confirm or dispel this notion, knowing that Maltz indicated it takes *at least* twenty-one days to form a habit. In her article published in the *European Journal of Social Psychology*, she conducted a study that examined the habits of ninety-six people over a twelve-week period. Each person picked one new habit and reported whether or not they performed the action and if it felt automatic. At the end of the twelve-week period, the findings were analyzed and then published. Lally found that, on average, it takes sixty-six days for a new behavior to become a habit. However, the exact time is based on the person, the type of behavior, environmental conditions, etc. Additionally, the researchers found that "missing one opportunity to perform the behavior did not materially affect the habit formation process."

So what does this have to do with abundance?

This truth is that, in terms of radical abundance, the role of consistency is to create a behavior of visualization and goal setting that becomes so normal it evolves into a habit because positive habits promote enormous abundance. The research above provides us with uplifting and exciting scientific support for the creation of abundance. It shows that:

1. If given the time, any behavior can become a habit. The science supports the notion that it does not call for a miracle to change the way you act or perceive the world.

2. It really doesn't take that long to create a habit. The research varies, but it could take as little as twenty-one days to two months to form a positive habit.

3. Finally, don't stress if you miss a day. Habits do require time and attention, but do not quit just because you are inconsistent in your road to consistency.

Habits do require consistency, but research supports the uplifting proposition that a small amount of dedicated time over a manageable period can create the essential behavior needed to manifest consistency and abundance within your life. Just like when you set goals, habits are formed through bite size chunks. That is how we've been trained. Sometimes you adopt limiting beliefs, ones that drag you down to the bottom of the pond. They may even occur at a very young age. The behaviors cause you to push the ball up the hill, rather than enjoying the momentum of rolling down the hill with it. Somewhere in your life lies a fault line or crack within your belief system that you have adopted as a truth. Until you unearth that belief system, until you know that the weed is in the garden, and until you choose to pull that weed up and cast it aside, you'll continue the behavior that is in direct opposition of consistency, supportive habits, and abundance.

You may be reading this and saying, "I don't know what beliefs are stopping me." We felt that same way, but we decided to check ourselves to defend against these greedy little joy eaters. These beliefs are like negative Pac-Men eating away at our hope, dreams, and vision. Well, you just need to get in the driver's seat again and understand that you are the only person who can control your thoughts. You are totally in charge. That's a change. You have the freedom to choose the thoughts with which you will dance, dine, and sleep. It's up to you. And yes it takes consistency.

You can go outside. You can listen to as many people as you want. You can do as much as you desire. But until you choose to own a different belief, and focus the time and energy on creating consistency in positive habits, you'll remain stagnant. In the beginning it may not even feel like it's your belief, but you have to own it and be with it enough that it becomes natural. That desire to own your belief inevitably leads to the action of consistent dedication to changing or adopting it. It is your responsibility to take control of your life and your behavior.

Life is filled with peaks and canyons, some over which we have little control. But we have a choice in how we surmount the peaks and navigate the canyons. So long as we are dedicated to personal consistency in our actions, we can overcome that which stands in the way. And we can welcome in a level of abundance that supports all we desire.

Radical Recap:

To ensure you create Radically Consistent results in your behavior, remember to:

1. Remain consistent in your visualization exercises, always focusing on that which you desire.
2. Set realistic goals and work to obtain them on a daily basis.
3. Commit to putting time and energy behind the results you want to create.
4. Never abandon the idea that success is yours for the taking.

Chapter 22:
RADICAL RESULTS

We do what we do to get results. Simple as that. In every aspect of our lives, our decisions and behaviors are always motivated by the need to secure a specific result. Whether those results are in the form of skincare or life-care, we apply a regiment, a prescription of sorts, so that we can turn one trajectory and direction into a better one. There is nothing more exciting than securing those results for which we aim, and substantially changing outcomes. But for change, we would fall short of growth. To begin our journey, we outlined a prescription, one that could help you to locate meaningful difference. Each step of that prescription keeps moving us closer and closer to the destination. And here we are at destiny's door, key in hand, ready to insert it and jar that door open.

Heraclitus was a Pre-Socratic Greek Philosopher. As most with philosophers, he subscribed to a rock-solid belief system. The foundation of that system was his almost ceaseless insistence on ever-present change as the fundamental essence of the universe. By that, he meant that to live we have to change. Change is the one certain in life. To that end, he proclaimed, "Big results require big ambitions." If you want to really make a difference, you have to decisively begin to dream at remarkable levels.

Throughout this book, we have worked to fan your fire of change. Mostly because a little bit of energy can go a long way. It's a basic prescription to create a not so basic life. We can get by with just enough. But just enough is not nearly as fulfilling. Our commitment is to illuminate the abundance that you deserve.

In short, we want to help *you* get results. Results in life, results in love, results in attitude, results in perception, and results in happiness. As you apply our prescription to your life you will see changes. We all strive for abundance: abundance in love, in happiness, in success, in friendships, in our profession, and in our financial security. Abundance is an exciting proposition. Throughout this book, we applied the metaphor of skincare to our lives. Our hope is that through this metaphor you can see the essential value in choosing the ingredients that are right for you to create a meaningful and super-effective regimen.

A Radical Reminder:

1. Say the Radical Yes – you'll never know when opportunity knocks.
2. Recognize the potential in adversity – it is always present.
3. Understand your beliefs – and rewrite them to serve you.
4. Decisions lead to outcomes – don't be afraid to make them.
5. Identify your passion and purpose – success and joy lives there.
6. Visualize the outcome you desire – imagine big and see it with emotion.
7. Set Goals – write them down in the present tense, be specific and read them often.
8. Embrace opportunity – it is there for you.
9. Build a team that supports your dream – they are your gift and you are theirs.
10. Be a difference maker – because you can.
11. Welcome in Abundance – consistently set goals, attract outcomes, and visualize dreams.

Within each of us is opportunity – the opportunity to awaken and welcome in radical abundance. It takes time, it calls for energy, and it requires nurturing, love, and attention.

When we asked successful people the key to happiness and success, we learned of many ingredients, including: ownership, goal setting, planning, leadership, hard work, knowledge, focus, commitment, passion, resilience, and many more. We learned that while knowledge and hard work come out high on the list, nothing overrides the attitude and passion that gives you the will to do it.

Through it all, we recognized that it's your attitude and not your altitude that determines how high you will fly in life. How high do you want to fly? Henry Ford said, "Whether you think that you can or not, you are right." So now we turn to you. Are you ready? Are you willing? We know you are able. This is your world and this is your life. You have the utmost responsibility and gift to turn your time on this earth into something so extremely meaningful that you become the radical light that illuminates the lives of others.

Chapter 23:
THE RADICAL REALITY

Use it or lose it. No pain, no gain. No time like the present. It's yours for the taking. The buck stops here. It's yours to win or lose. You get out of it what you put into it. Put up or shut up. Today is the first day of the rest of your life. It's all in your mind. You are what you eat. Like attracts like. Age is nothing but a number. Live in the moment. The past is in the past. That which does not kill us makes us stronger. The darkest hour is just before the dawn. One step at a time. Keep the faith. Stretch. Actions speak louder than words. Birds of a feather flock together. Count your blessings. History repeats itself. If a job is worth doing it is worth doing well. If at first you don't succeed then try, try and try again. It's better to give than to receive. It's never too late. Never put off until tomorrow what you can do today. Practice makes perfect. Where there's a will there's a way. It takes a village. To be or not to be. Actions speak louder than words.

How many times have we heard the above? If you are like most of us, the answer is: for as long as we can remember. Each of these clichés leads us to the radical reality that Radical Action is a prerequisite to reach your heart's greatest desires. Change is required. A supportive belief system is required. Setting goals and visualizing are required. And the only person that can decide to accomplish each of these is you. That is the Radical Reality.

History will repeat itself, especially if you keep living your life the same way and do not decide to invest the hard work and dedication it takes to be better. The tools that you have read about, the principles in this book, are fresh in your mind, and practice does actually make perfect. Use it or lose it. If you don't use the tools and principles that you have learned, you will lose the opportunity to see extraordinary results. You only have this moment. The power is truly in the present. The power is in you. You're the only person that can create the results that you want.

Think about this moment in your life. Consider where you are. Now recognize that which you desire can be yours. A radical life you love requires a radical approach: Not accepting the unacceptable and pushing the boundaries of your mind to believe and achieve what you really want for your life. The power to have all that your heart desires is within you. This book has given you the tools, the direction, and the course. But none of that really matters unless you Get Radical and use them. It is up to you.

It is really just a game of inches. One step at a time, one prescriptive measure after another, you will begin to see the difference that radical creates. So why not you? So why not now? We are committed to the notion that it is possible to love your skin again, just as it is possible to regain love for your life. You just need to get radical in your approach. You are now part of our Radical Dream Team. You have had Radical Access to transformational ingredients and formulas that make a radical difference. Your happiness and fulfillment will be part of our legacy becoming a reality. The warmth and motivation you provide others through burning bright is what our world needs. If we all work to be the light for one another, to share these radical principles, and to join together on this life-changing journey, we will all have the opportunity to be empowered and inspired to live radical lives that we love.

We wrote this book to be your lantern and to guide you through the dark corners and unknowns of your journey. Embracing all of our perfect imperfections together, we hope to give you the light that has helped to illuminate our path. But like any lantern, it is now our time to pass the torch and light yours. Take great care of your potential. You are the light. You have the ability to burn bright. You are the reason we created Radical Skincare. You are the reason we took the last three years to write *Get Radical.* Now, you are the best person to write the next chapter. The chapter of your life begins today. Your success and fulfillment are the next part of our journey. So turn the page and write your chapter like your life depends on it. We continue to hear our parent's words: "To be the difference you must make a difference." Our hope is that we have done a bit of that with this book.

We thank you for your generous spirit and time to take this journey with us.

Now it's your turn to *Get Radical.*

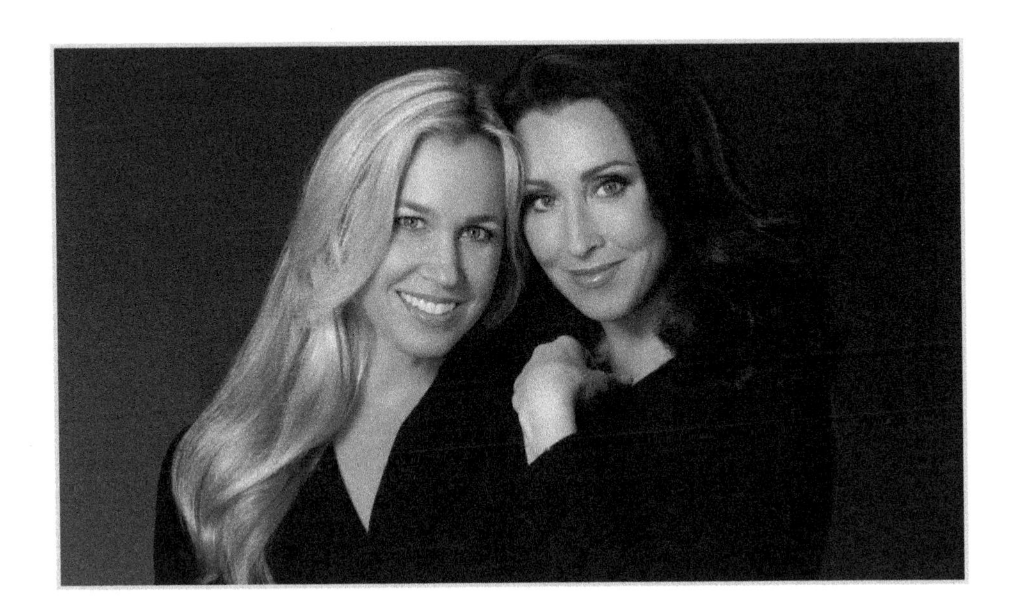

ABOUT THE AUTHORS

From a very young age, their parents always told the Edlich sisters: 'To be the difference you must make a difference." Throughout their lives, this mantra burned within them. Growing up on a farm in Charlottesville Virginia, Liz and Rachel developed their work ethic from the most fundamental levels as they embraced the essence of life in its most basic manner. Whether it is the world of non-profit, investment banking or the challenges of entrepreneurship, they carry the innate compassion to understand how creative brilliance and adversity can live side by side.

The road was not always easy. They witnessed their parents struggle with degenerative diseases and watched their family get torn apart through the obstacles that were simply too burdensome. But they took these difficult lessons and used them to fuel personal growth and development.

It was through this everlasting desire to evolve that the two sisters became business partners and created Radical Skincare. It became their purpose; it was their calling. As they created a formula for skincare, they realized within it was a prescription for life. Their hope is that *Get Radical* and the lessons shared herein, by some of their exceptional mentors and friends, will make a difference in each of your lives, and contribute to helping you create the life that you love no matter what adversities you may encounter.

www.RadicalSkincare.com

Notes

1 http://www.everydayhealth.com/rosacea/rosacea-basics.aspx
2 http://www.medicaldaily.com/facts-skin-aging-240955
3 https://www.changingfaces.org.uk/show/feature/NEWS-look-at-me-prelim-report
4 http://unstoppablefoundation.org/about-us/
5 http://www.ideastogo.com/the-science-of-imagination
6 http://www.ideastogo.com/the-science-of-imagination
7 http://www.forbes.com/sites/lisaquast/2011/10/31/how-becoming-a-mentor-can-boost-your-career/
8 http://www.pickthebrain.com/blog/15-fascinating-facts-about-smiling/
9 http://www.pickthebrain.com/blog/15-fascinating-facts-about-smiling/
10 https://www.brucelipton.com/books/biology-of-belief
11 http://life.gaiam.com/article/power-friendship
12 http://www.etymonline.com/index.php?term=courage
13 http://www.biography.com/people/tippi-hedren-9333313#life-off-screen
14 http://www.livestrong.com/article/135849-what-are-benefits-self-confidence/
15 Lorna Vanderhaeghe, MS: CHFA West, presentation notes
16 http://www.irishexaminer.com/lifestyle/healthandlife/yourhealth/the-ugly-truth-why-women-arent-happy-with-their-looks-245111.html
17 http://www.boredpanda.com/love-facts-list/
18 http://www.boredpanda.com/love-facts-list/
19 http://www.forbes.com/2009/12/22/volunteering-community-service-corporate-responsibility-forbes-woman-leadership-nethope.html
20 http://www.huffingtonpost.com/vanessa-van-edwards/the-science-of-goal-setting_b_6335764.html
21 [24] Ibid.
[25] Ibid.
22 [26] http://stroke.ahajournals.org/content/38/4/1293.short
23 [27] http://www.huffingtonpost.com/james-clear/forming-newhabits_b_5104807.html

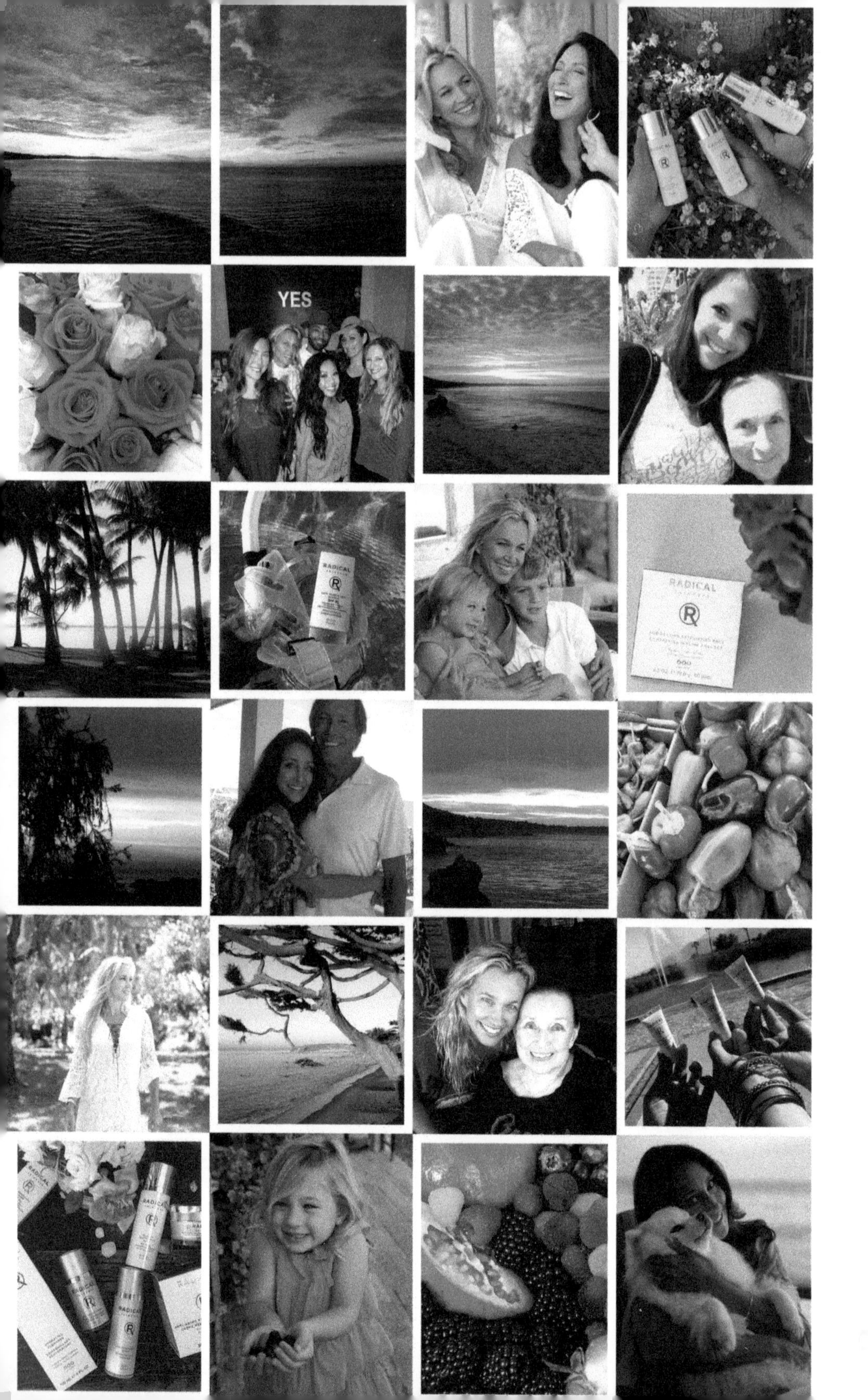
YES
RADICAL